About the author

Frank Navratil Bsc. N.D. was born of Czech parents in Vancouver, Canada where he completed a degree in physiology and nutrition. In the 1990's he moved to Sydney, Australia where he studied alternative medicine and iridology before practicing as a naturopath, iridologist, and nutritionist. Since 1997, he has lived in Prague, the Czech Republic where he currently runs a natural therapy practice, produces an alternative medicine Internet magazine, and directs a school offering courses in alternative medicine.

Frank has given countless lectures both in the Czech Republic and in Australia on the subject of iris diagnosis and nutrition. He has also appeared on several television and radio programs to talk about natural means of diagnosing and dealing with disease. He is the author of a number or article series on iris diagnosis and nutrition that have been published in alternative medicine and health magazines in Australia and the Czech Republic.

He has worked, too, in Ethiopia where he studied the effects of malnutrition and he is presently cooperating with an Ethiopian Aid agency to fund the development of an Education Center for the prevention of disease there.

His practice is based on natural holistic methods that allow the body to heal itself. These include iridology, nutrition, vitamin and mineral treatment, Bowen therapy, and diet and lifestyle changes.

FOR YOUR EYES ONLY

A Fascinating Look at the Art and Science of Iris Diagnosis,
the Diagnostic Method of the New Millennium.

Frank Navratil BSc. N.D.

Published by Frank Navratil, BSc. N.D.
Kojetická 977, Neratovice
Prague
Czech Republic
First Edition
Cover photographs by Petra Růžičková
All eye photographs by Frank Navratil, BSc. N.D.
© 2001 by Frank Navratil

ISBN 80-238-7220-6

CONTENTS

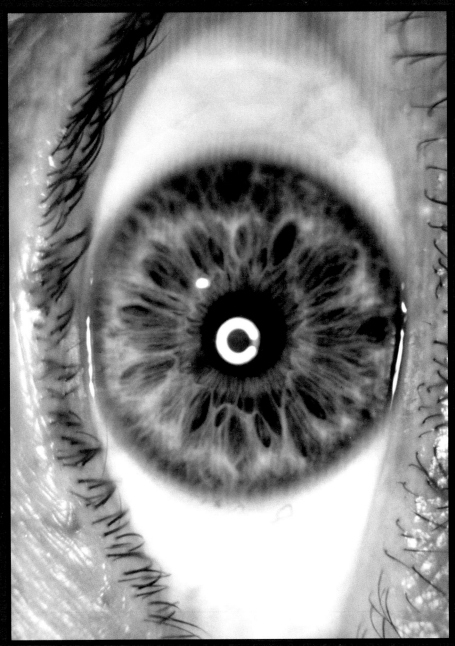

"Nature has bestowed upon us the most magnificent diagnostic tools that modern medical science could ever imagine, our eyes"

Preface

The beauty of simplicity

What do we mean when we refer to the word, "simple"? Generally, we mean something that is not difficult, is easy, uncomplicated and without stress. Sometimes we refer to "simple" as something that is available to everyone, not only to the well educated, or to the rich and famous.

When I lived in Australia before settling down in my new home, the Czech Republic, I would often gaze upon the vast blue ocean beaches and contemplate the deep truth, that it is the simplest things in life that bring us the most happiness. I would watch wave after wave come crashing towards the shore as I pondered how nature always seemed to bring us back to the realization of what is really important in life. I couldn't help but wonder why we as mankind are so intent upon complicating our lives.

In modern times we have destroyed much of what is natural around us. We have forgotten that we as human beings have to interact with our natural environment, since our world is an endless transfer of energy from one medium to another. We have closed ourselves off in a world full of low-energy, man-made computer technology, unhealthy working conditions, and modern stress that our early ancestors never had to endure. Our fast-paced lifestyles have created greater nutritional demands on our bodies. Ignoring that need, we fill our stomachs with fast food and instant preparations full of chemical additives as we constantly search for complicated solutions to our growing health problems. Do you know that statistically we are less healthy than we were 60 years ago? Yes, we are perhaps living longer than we did a hundred years ago, but are we living a quality life? Do we even know what a quality healthy life is? Certainly it is not one that involves several bouts of flu every year, or the feeling of chronic fatigue where we have to drag ourselves up every morning to go to work. It certainly doesn't mean that our back and joints ache or that our head often hurts, or that we get out of breath every time we climb a short flight of stairs. A quality healthy life surely doesn't mean that at the end of the working day we barely have enough energy left to watch TV and fall into bed.

A quality healthy life is rare these days, but simply like a sunset or the cascading ocean waves, it is available to most of us. All we need to do is to open our eyes and return to a natural way of life.

Our modern world has forced us to grow accustomed to taking drugs for every common ailment. However, we have not been made to understand that we cannot fool our bodies by man-made preparations with frequently dangerous side effects; we can only fool ourselves. Mankind has invented a variety of complicated methods to diagnose disease, including x-rays, CAT scans, blood tests, electrocardiographs, and a number of technologically sophisticated tests. Patients undergoing them are often placed through time-consuming, often painful, and sometimes hazardous procedures to determine what disease they really have. Every year companies search for technology that promises to diagnose a disease more accurately and they invest millions of dollars in research. However, I have found in my practice with patients that many had often endured endless tests with absolutely no results, or the disease had been diagnosed but the root of the disease remained unknown.

Surprisingly, we already have at our disposal the most naturally sophisticated tool for diagnosing not just disease, but most importantly, the causes of disease. It is something that almost all of us possess, our eyes. Yes, it is these magnificent organs that allow us not only to view the world around us, but that also act as a map to every organ, gland, and system in our body.

It is because of my strong belief in and passion for iridology, the art and science of diagnosing health status from what is seen in the iris, pupil, and sclera of the eyes, that I am sharing this book with you. I thank the thousands of patients whose eyes I have photographed over several years for allowing me to accumulate enough research material to base this book upon. Welcome to an intriguing world and a fascinating branch of alternative medicine. In my opinion, iris diagnosis is the only real method I know of that at a glance can provide me with a wonderfully true picture of a patient's entire health status. Iris diagnosis has helped a great many patients learn more about their state of health and what to do to make improvements.

This book is for everyone, including health professionals who want to investigate making diagnosis from the eyes. I hope you enjoy the book and learn from it, but most of all I hope it will inspire you and provide you with an alternative outlook on how health can be viewed in the human body.

Remember, the eyes are not only the windows to our souls; they are hidden maps to our bodies.

This book is dedicated to the beauty of simplicity, which inspired it; for in every complicated array of problems there is often just a simple solution, or an unsophisticated answer. We just have to open our eyes. This is the beauty of simplicity.

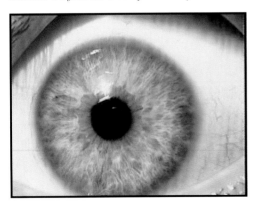

Frank Navratil BSc. N.D.

6

My Beliefs

- I believe that iris diagnosis is the most precise form of diagnosis that exists and as more research is made on it, it may become the method of choice of diagnosis in the future.

- I believe that what is seen in the eyes in the form of colors, marks or specific signs is representative of degenerative changes that are occurring in specific organs of the body.

- I believe that changes in the eyes occur along with changes in health status.

- I believe that iris diagnosis is not designed to label a disease, but to find the root or cause of the condition.

- I believe that chemical drugs may alleviate the symptoms of a disease, but will not cure it.

- I believe that we must look at all aspects of health to remedy illness. This includes the physical, the psychological, and the spiritual.

- I believe that foods should only be consumed in their natural form.

- I believe that we must not alter our food supply either chemically or genetically.

- I believe that poor nutrition and stress are the basis of the majority of health problems.

- I believe in natural vitamins and food supplements to assist health or prevent disease in our modern society as the quality of food in recent times has declined.

- I believe that without regular exercise, one cannot achieve optimum health.

- I believe that physical health status influences psychological behavior and vice versa.

- I believe that ninety percent of health problems today are due to improper diet and lifestyle decisions.

- I believe in iris diagnosis and alternative medicine as they focus on natural methods of diagnosing health problems and improving the state of health of the individual so that the body can heal itself.

Acknowledgements

I would like to thank my mother, Ludmila Navratil, whose lengthy illness and death from cancer several years ago, motivated me to become interested in alternative medicine and iridology.

I would also like to thank all my past patients for their belief and support as from them, I have learned a great deal about iridology. Their eyes have given me an abundance of research material so that I could write and share what I had learned.

I would like to thank all the iridologists of the past who have inspired me to continue in this great science and who have permitted me to learn and expand upon their pioneering work.

I would like to thank Hanka Kopecká for her love, patience and support while I labored at the time-consuming task of writing this book.

I would like to thank Mr. and Mrs. Kopecký of Hnátnice, Czech Republic for the use of their country home where I wrote most of this book.

I would like to thank Dr. Bernard Jensen who inspired me to believe that the body can heal itself through nutrition.

Chapter 1

Introduction: The eyes are not just the windows to the soul

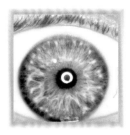

"Often as we travel, we come across several obstacles in our lives or crossroads that present to us a variety of directions to take. There is no right or wrong direction if we listen to our intuition and to our heart."

When people are asked what they look at first when they notice an attractive person, several answers come to mind. Some say they observe how a person walks or what he or she is wearing. Some detect the perfume or cologne they wear, some take in the body type, or the color and style of hair. However, a great proportion of people first notice the eyes of a person, for the eyes are often described as the windows to the soul. When we look into people's eyes, we can often determine whether they are lying, whether they are angry or whether they are in love. We often can tell whether people are tired or not feeling well because eyes appear dull and lack the usual sparkle when people are not in the best of health. However, the eye is not only the window to our soul; the eye is also a map to our body.

Welcome on a journey that will take you to destinations where perhaps you have never been before and through experiences that may change the way you have thought about health and medicine in the past. It is always a risk to be open to new ideas but I know the risk and the journey will be well worth taking.

I would like to introduce to you a diagnostic method that belongs under the branch of alternative medicine and called iridology or as it is commonly known, iris diagnosis. This method involves diagnosis of one's state of health by specific colors, marks, and signs that are seen in the iris of the eyes. I, however, like to think of iris diagnosis as not just a study of the iris, but also the pupil and sclera which often reveal a number of other significant health problems.

Have you ever noticed that there frequently appear clouds or marks in the iris of your eye and that these change depending on the state of your health or age? Have you noticed that your left eye is different from your right eye? If you have, I congratulate you, as many people believe that their eye color remains the same in both eyes all of their lives.

After studying thousands and thousands of irises in great detail over many years, I have had the opportunity to notice several changes in the irises, pupils, and sclera of eyes and have come to the conclusion that what is revealed in the eyes, mirrors the state of health of our entire body. That's right, the iris of the eye is actually a map where each place represents a different body organ or system.

But first, before I try to convince those of you who may be unsure or skeptical about this method, I would like to discuss the terms "individuality" and "holistic medicine," both of which are very close to my heart.

You are not Normal

What do we mean by normal? Is anyone out there really normal? Normality is something that we have contrived and refers to anything that does not deviate from a norm or average value. We are constantly bombarded with normal values, such as normal height, normal weight, and normal body temperature. We all know what normal behavior is according to society norms and if we deviate from this behavior we often are classified as crazy. In modern times there are norms for everything, including norms for every kind of medical symptom or classification of health status. Is this a rational way to look at a human being or are we sometimes forgetting the one plain fact that distinguishes us from any other person, the fact that we are not normal?

Yes, that is right, each one of us is special, an individual with different needs and attributes. It is often a mistake to look at an individual using normal values because each of us has a different liver, a different ability to dispose of toxins in the body, a different metabolism, a different ability to handle stress, and a different need for nutrients. How then can a drug, for example, be prescribed for every single patient using a normal dosage? We are often reminded of this error since a dosage of a drug given to one person may cause stomach upset or side effects, while the same dosage given to another patient causes no reaction at all. Each one of us is different. No expert in the world can predict what a combination of several drugs will do to our body as each of us has different abilities to deal with the drugs. This poses a great danger as the body is being put through an experiment each time because no matter how many times a drug has been tested on people, every single person is a new experiment. Do you want to persist in allowing drugs to experiment with your body?

I believe that each one of us is unique. No one is superior to another, just different. As we learn about our bodies and ourselves, we grow to appreciate that we are not normal; that each of us is an individual. Iris diagnosis appreciates this simple fact of individuality. Every iris is different. Like a fingerprint or a tongue print it distinguishes us from any other person. Using iris diagnosis, one can view each patient as an individual and in many cases can uncover the unique strengths and weaknesses that make us who we are.

Holistic Health

I believe that in order to really understand the value of iris diagnosis, one must understand the concept of holistic health. This term is often used in alternative medicine but its main premise is to view the body as a whole rather than as only specific parts. This is quite rational because each of our cells, each of our organs, and each of our systems, all interact together.

When one organ in the body is not functioning well, the whole body is affected. Modern medicine often fails because specialization in a specific area often neglects this fact and therefore the root of the problem remains.

Alternative medicine seeks to analyze total health or holistic health and this includes more than just the physical. Psychological health and spiritual health are also considered important in getting to the root of the patient's health problems.

Take for example, a patient with skin problems. He or she may focus only on the skin and search endlessly for ointments, skin lotions and skin preparations but is the skin really the core of the problem? Often the real core of the problem lies with one of our cleansing organs, which may include the intestines, the liver, the kidneys or the lungs. Perhaps it is stress that is creating a mineral or vitamin deficiency. The core of the problem may then be one of psychological health and may reflect a current stressful situation or past psychological scars. Do you see where I am going now? Holistic health includes all areas that affect our health status. The doctors of the future will have to take all aspects of health into consideration if they want to successfully cure their patients and this leads me to another question. When you receive a drug prescription for a medical problem you may have, do you feel that you are treated or cured? There is a big difference. If you are only treated, it means that the condition periodically recurs or shows up as something else even a few years later. With every chemical drug there is a side effect. That means that some part of the body suffers as a result of the treatment. For example taking heavy doses of antibiotics often leads to destruction of beneficial micro flora in the intestines, leading to all sorts of medical problems in the future. Is that holistic health? It certainly is not! It is only a fast and irresponsible way of dealing with a medical problem which does not take into account the effects it will have on the whole body. I say to all my patients that there is no fast, miraculous way to return to health. It takes work and lifestyle changes. Holistic health is the only health that I believe in.

If you now understand a little about holistic health you will see how iris diagnosis is related. Iris diagnosis is the only diagnostic method I know that allows one to view all the interacting systems and organs and how they affect each other. In my opinion, it is the diagnostic method of the future. Just think, all that information encoded in your irises, which are each just a few millimeters in diameter.

Rationale for the theory of Iris diagnosis

You may be asking - how can the iris of the eye reflect conditions in our body? This is a very reasonable question and I was very skeptical when first introduced to the concept that information in the form of certain signs encoded in the iris can reflect our state of health. But is this really such a bizarre and crazy idea? Think for a moment. We can often recognize an unhealthy person when we see one. How do we know he is unhealthy?

Perhaps, we notice his poor skin color or condition, excessive perspiration, unhealthy hair, or glazed, weak and tired eyes.

Those are all signs the body reveals, that tell us something is not working right. In the same way, the iris of our eyes displays colors and marks when something is not right in the body. So let's take the assumption that if our bodies are not healthy, certain marks or colors appear in the irises of the eyes. Now, this of course doesn't mean that a mark in a certain place in the iris represents a kidney problem. How can we be sure? We can't, but through experience with thousands and thousands of patients who have had the same kidney problem, it has been found that they had similar marks in generally the same place in the iris.

A possible scientific explanation is that the eyes are connected by the nervous system via the optic nerve to our brain. Many believe that the brain records information on every physical and psychological event that occurs in our bodies. If the eye is connected to this human computer we call the brain, it is reasonable to hypothesize that colors and marks in the eyes change in response to changes in our bodies and are recorded in similar places just like the human brain has certain areas that record and retain information.

Through my iris studies, I have confirmed these occurrences time and time again. However, I may be convinced but that doesn't mean that you are.

Another piece of scientific information that might interest you is that the eyeball is not really a smooth surface. When viewed closely under a microscope the surface of the iris is one of hills and valleys and the areas that we see as dark spots on the iris are in actual fact crevices or deeper layers of the eye, while white spots are actually raised areas on the iris. Generally iridologists believe that the greater the degeneration of the organ, the darker the corresponding area on the iris. Again, I have confirmed this occurrence many times as seen in tumors showing up as deep dark areas on the iris.

Another question that has been posed to those in the modern medical field is why do colors in the irises of the eyes change and why are the colors and marks different in the left and right eyes? So far, there has been no real scientific explanation and there needs to be more research conducted to validate the method of iris diagnosis so that it can become accepted by modern medicine.

There are also other factors that have contributed to the support of the theory of iridology such as the fact that past iris maps that had been developed in different countries consistently showed remarkable similarities even though they were developed independently of each other.

As modern technology and computers develop more inroads into the fascinating world of iridology, I am sure that even more accurate iris maps will evolve and what thousands of iridologists have always known will finally be generally accepted. I know of only one country, Russia that has come close to accepting iris diagnosis into modern medicine. Currently, the greatest amount of research on iris diagnosis is being done in countries such as Germany, Australia, and America, as well as Russia.

History of Iridology

A book on iridology would not be complete without at least a brief look at how mankind first came to use this method.

We do not know exactly when man first discovered a correlation between parts of the body and the iris of the eye, but we do know that even the ancient Chaldeans had entertained this concept. The first record in history is from the year 1690 when Phillipe Meyens in Dresden published the book "Chiromatica Medica". The book described how the top part of the iris represents the head and the lower part represents the kidneys, spleen and genital organs. Also it was then first recognized that the left side of the iris corresponds to the left side of the body and the right side of the iris, the right side of the body.

A few other publications had been made, but it was not until the early 1800's that iridology had its official beginning in the modern era. One very remarkable person and one very remarkable incident changed the face of what we know as iridology today.

That person was Ignatz von Peczely, born in Hungary in 1826, who at the age of 11 accidentally broke the leg of an owl while attempting to let it free from his garden. He noticed that in the lower part of the owl's eye there appeared a black stripe. After he splinted the owl's leg and allowed a period of time for it to heal, white lines appeared where the dark line had been before.

The bird stayed with him in the garden for several years where he had time to notice the changes that occurred in the iris of the owl's eye.

That amazing experience made a lasting impression on the young Peczely and later in his career as a homeopathic physician he had the opportunity to study the eyes of his patients in great detail and was able to confirm his diagnoses by performing several autopsies. He began to diagnose from the eye and soon became famous all over the country. He was accused many times of fraud by the medical profession of the time, who saw his technique as a form of witchcraft. It often seems to me that not much has changed in 150 years as I myself constantly come across people who view iridology as charlatanry and even to this date iridology in many countries in the world is banned or ridiculed by the classical medical profession. However, it does continue to thrive and recently there has been renewed interest in this method all around the world. I believe that eventually, it will be used to support the methods that we currently use. A change for the good is always a difficult, but rewarding road.

In 1880 Von Peczely published his only book called " Discoveries in the Realms of Nature and Art of Healing," and in 1886 the first iridology map of the eye was revealed for the world to see. Today, Ignatz von Peczely is known as the father of iridology and his studies continue to inspire the many great iridologists who have followed his path to our modern history.

Other notable iridologists soon emerged like Nils Liljequist from Stockholm, Sweden who discovered that color changes occur in the iris of the eye.

Iridology later spread to the United States when Dr. Henry Lane from Germany began doing work in Illinois and published his findings in 1904.

One of Lane's students, Dr. Henry Lindlahr went on to promote and study iridology. His monumental work was published in 1913.

Dr. Bernard Jensen, who is recognized as the leading iridologist in the United States, studied with Lindlahr in the early nineteen twenties.

Meanwhile, in Germany and Europe, iridology was moving forward with prominent iridologists like Dr. Rudolf Schnabel, Joseph Angerer, Theodore Kriege, and Josef Deck who have contributed immensely to this profession.

After the Second World War, iris diagnosis took a great leap forward, as an estimated ten thousand medical doctors began to study and use iris diagnosis as their primary diagnostic tool. Unfortunately, the German medical association had often made attempts to ban those practicing natural therapy and iridology and thus, the number of practitioners, greatly decreased. It seems that iridology has always had a rocky road, but the fact that it has endured for over 200 years is indicative of its lasting value. It is only a matter of time, I believe, before computers and modern technology confirm iris findings and finally, scientifically prove this phenomenon. Then it will assuredly become widely accepted by the medical community.

Today, iridology is used all over the world not only in Germany or the United States, but also in many countries including Spain, Portugal, Australia, England and Russia. I do hope that this book will inspire many others to bring iridology to the forefront of modern medicine.

Chapter 2

Genetic Iris Constitutions

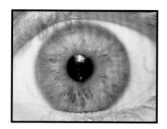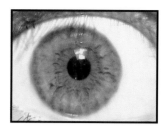

"To some extent our health depends on what we inherit genetically. This is what makes each one of us different from one another."

Do we genetically inherit traits from our parents or great grandparents?

Can we see these genetic characteristics when we look at the iris of the eye?

Can we predict what level of health an individual has or will have by what we see in the eyes?

The answer is, " yes " to the above questions. First, we need to understand a little about grades of iris fiber density and then we can determine our genetic iris constitution.

Grades of Iris Fiber Density

When we look closely at an iris through a microscope we see that it is composed of fibers that run radially outward from the pupil. In some eyes these fibers are closely packed together and in others they are packed very loosely. This is a very important characteristic determining the strength of the genetic constitution. I like to look initially at the iris fiber density because it immediately gives the general genetic strength of the patient. I use a grading system of 5 levels with Grade A being the genetically strongest and Grade E, the weakest.

A **Grade A** iris is very rarely seen. It belongs to a perfectly healthy individual with iris fibers closely and densely packed together, where the color of the iris is uniform and no sign of breaks in the fibers or discoloration is found.

A **Grade B** iris is also not very often seen. It belongs to an individual who seldom has any medical problems although with advancing years some problems may become evident. The color is consistent within the iris but the fibers begin to show a looser structure.

A **Grade C** iris is the most commonly seen. It belongs to an individual who is more prone to disease. The iris structure includes discoloration, clouds, pigment deposits, or lacunae (breaks in iris fibers). Often there are deformities in the radial fibers.

A **Grade D** iris has only loosely packed fibers as well as clouds, lacunae, uneven coloring, pigments and fibers that often run transverse rather than radial. These individuals usually have metabolic problems, are over-acidic and have difficulty eliminating waste products from the body. People with this grade of iris often suffer from liver, kidney, back and muscular problems.

A **Grade E** iris has all the above, but the border around the ruff zone (zone that encircles the pupil) is becoming uneven and the outer ring of the iris darkened. There are gaps between fibers and sometimes the fibers cannot be seen. Various defects in the iris become apparent and can extend from the pupil right to the outer part of the iris. These individuals have hormonal and metabolic problems and a deteriorating nervous system. These patients will require constant treatment during their lives.

Eye pictures of different grades

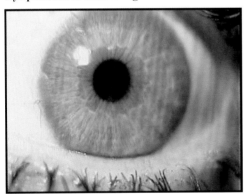

Grade B

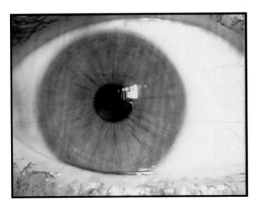

Grade C

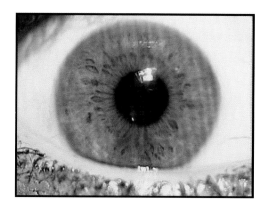

Grade D

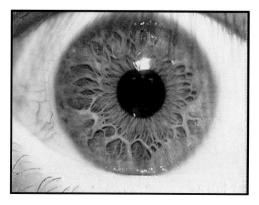

Grade E

Introduction to Iris Constitutions

As I have already mentioned, we are all individuals and each of our eyes is unique but through studies of thousands of irises, a number of genetic types or constitutions appear to exist. This does not in any way detract from the fact that our eyes are all different. It only allows classification of types of eyes that are most commonly seen in the world today. Every eye is unique but there are general similarities among many types of eyes.

When we refer to our genetic constitution, we mean, "what we are made of," our strengths and weaknesses and those attributes we have inherited from our parents, grandparents, etc.

Studies in iridology have revealed that there exist a number of constitutions or similar types of eyes each with its own physical and psychological characteristics. Each of us is born with a genetic iris constitution. Knowing not only the grade of fiber density but also the type of constitution can be very valuable as it identifies weaknesses and permits an understanding of potential health problems. In my studies of thousands of eyes, I have never come across a perfect iris. Each one of us has certain weaknesses, some of which do not become evident until later in life. While we cannot change our constitution, we can influence the constitution in a positive or a negative way. This in turn will affect the passing on of traits to our offspring.

Studies on dogs have shown that it takes three generations of vitamin therapy and quality nutrition to perceive a genetic trait completely disappear. This means that what we inherit may not have to be something that is passed on to our future generations. We need to start improving our lifestyles so that the coming generations are not plagued with medical and health problems.

Some of the numerous negative influences that can cause a weakened genetic constitution include: inadequate nutrition, too much alcohol, shock, physical or mental trauma, hunger, pollution and smog, drugs, cigarette smoking, depression, stress, radiation, lack of exercise, lack of sunlight, obesity, chemical poisoning and many other factors.

Positive influences that strengthen our genetic constitution include: living in a clean natural environment, quality nutrition, regular exercise, fresh air and sunlight, natural medicine without the use of drugs, good moral behavior, positive thoughts and actions, a balance between friends, family and work, the emotional, spiritual and material, and the ability to accept ourselves as we are.

Genotype And Phenotype

Our health is influenced by two factors, genotype and phenotype. Genotype refers to our genetic make-up or constitution, that which we are born with. These are the genetic iris constitutions, which will be described in detail in this chapter.

The phenotype is what we develop during our lives depending on the type of environment, our diet, and any physical or emotional events that we experience. Analyzing the phenotype of an individual through signs in the iris will be discussed in later chapters.

Our phenotype combines with our genotype to make us unique individuals along with unique susceptibilities to illness or health.

I have studied thousands of people with the following genetic iris constitutions and found that they have similar characteristics. There exist many other types, but I have found that these 10 are seen most often in my studies of eyes. Almost every individual's iris can be placed within one of these constitutional types. Knowing your genetic constitution is a very important step in developing an accurate diagnosis of your health status.

An understanding of your constitution will inspire or motivate you to make some positive changes for better health. Each one of you is special in your own way and deserves the best, so that you can achieve all the goals and dreams of your life. More about nutrition for individual genetic iris constitutions is found in my book, "The Eye for an Eye Diet."

Genetic iris constitutions:
1. Lymphatic Hyper-active
2. Lymphatic Hypo-active
3. Kidney Lymphatic
4. Neuro-Lymphatic
5. Hydro-Lymphatic
6. Hematogenic

7. Mixed
8. Plethoric
9. Hormonal
10. Connective Tissue

Each of these ten iris constitutions are presented individually and explained in detail.

Lymphatic Hyper-active

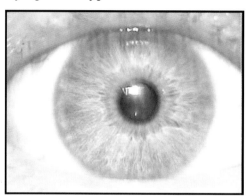

Physical Iris Description: a blue iris that may appear gray blue with closely compacted fiber density. Color is uniform and pigments are absent. A light rosary of clouds can be seen on the outer iris border as well as a white colored ruff zone and white around the ruff zone border.

General Complaints:

– Enlarged lymph nodes and congested lymphatic circulation
– Sensitive and over-reactive mucous membranes that often produce allergies in nose, throat, ear, and lung areas
– Allergies to milk lactose are common
– Weakness in the circulation, commonly felt as cold hands and feet
– All conditions generally improve with warmth
– Problems in the utilization of some vitamins, calcium, magnesium and iron

Common Complaints in Childhood:

– Eczema, skin rashes, hives, acne, and seborrhagic dermatitis
– Ear, nose, throat, tonsil and adenoid inflammation or infection
– Allergies and swollen glands
– Hyper-reactive mucous membranes causing respiratory conditions like bronchitis or asthma

Common Complaints in Adulthood:

– Childhood complaints may become chronic
– Excessive mucous production may result in discharges from the nose, ears and throat
– Inflammation of mucous membranes may cause respiratory problems like sinusitis, bronchitis and asthma
– Stiffness in joints and rheumatic and arthritic complaints
– Endocrine problems involving the parathyroid may cause problems like osteoporosis

–   Retention of fluids with depletion of energy
–   Congested and irritated lymphatic circulation resulting in swollen, painful glands

Lymphatic Hypo-reactive

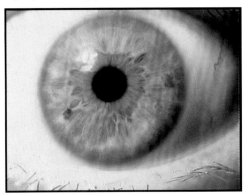

Physical Iris Description: a blue to blue-gray iris with other colors often seen in clouds or pigments in the iris, giving the eye a discolored and dull appearance. Many clouds are found in the outside ring of the iris connected by spoke-like runners from the center of the iris. These clouds are often yellow or brown. The center of the iris around the pupil, the ruff zone, is often a dirty brown color.

General Complaints:
–   Poor ability to eliminate waste products from the body
–   Under-active bowel, kidneys, liver, skin, respiratory organs, and lymphatic circulation
–   Poor elimination often leads to long-term stress on the heart and circulation
–   Mucous membranes tend to produce inadequate mucus, leading to irritation and inflammation
–   Generally slow recovery or regeneration from illness and injury

Common Complaints in Childhood:
–   Children with this constitution often look older than their age
–   Often weaknesses in the ear, nose and throat, tonsils, adenoids
–   Sensitive skin which may result in rashes
–   Due to frequent bacterial infections these children are often subjected to high antibiotic use which can lead to a compromised immune system and poor bowel function

Common Complaints in Adulthood:
–   Skin problems like eczema, psoriasis, boils, and fungal skin and nail infections are common due to the inability to eliminate waste products efficiently
–   Chronic inflammation of the mucous membranes and under-active lymphatic system and hardening of lymph nodes causing conditions like, tonsillitis, rhinitis, and discharge from ears and nose
–   Breath can be sour and foul body 'odor is common
–   Insufficient functioning of the liver and kidneys
–   Water retention leading to edema especially in the legs is common
–   Retention of toxins can also cause depression, or mood changes
–   Poor circulation in the veins and weaknesses in the heart
–   Arthritis due to drying out of tissues

   —   Reduction in activity of mucous membranes in the digestive system which can lead to reduced absorption and metabolism of vitamins and nutrients from the diet

Kidney Lymphatic

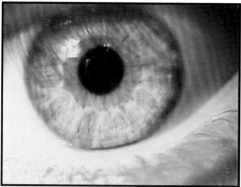

Physical Iris Description: a blue to blue gray iris with yellow around the ruff zone or yellow clouds around the outer iris giving the eye the appearance of being green. Occasionally, these yellow signs can be seen in a brown iris. The kidney area of the iris often displays defects or weakening signs.

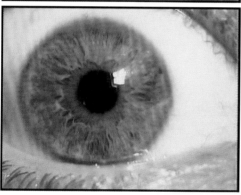

General Complaints:

   —   Genetically weakened kidneys which are stressed due to defective metabolism of proteins and foreign toxins often caused by a poor intake of fluids or too much of the wrong kind of fluids

   —   Dark "kidney bags" under the eyes during times when the kidneys are stressed, a fatty shine can also indicate liver involvement

   —   Tend not to feel thirsty, must be trained to drink more fluids

   —   Associated renal problems include edema, bladder infections, kidney stones and nephritis

   —   Sensitive mucous membranes especially around the ear, nose, throat, sinuses, and tonsils which can give rise to tonsillitis, bronchitis, and infections

   —   Prone to allergies like hay fever

   —   Skin is very sensitive and prone to skin rashes, itching skin, dry skin, or eczema

   —   Asthma is common

– Congestion of the lymphatic system
– Prone to headaches or migraines due to retention of fluid or accumulation of toxic substances in the blood
– Due to a predisposition to high levels of uric acid, rheumatoid and arthritic problems are commonly seen in older age
– Disposition to heart and circulation problems due to high levels of nitrogenous wastes in the blood

Common Complaints in Childhood:

– Children may have a very high sensitivity to skin rashes or eczema
– Inflammation of the mucous membranes
– Congestion of the lymphatic circulation
– Tonsillitis is commonly seen

Common Complaints in Adulthood:

– Insufficiency of the kidneys due to nephritis and edema
– Headaches or migraines
– Bladder infections
– Ear and sinus problems and hay fever
– Men often suffer from cramps or colic-type pain
– Liver complaints
– Rheumatoid arthritis and gout in old age due to the accumulation of uric acid
– Diseases of the heart and the circulatory system are often seen
– Great sensitivity to wetness and cold

Neurolymphatic

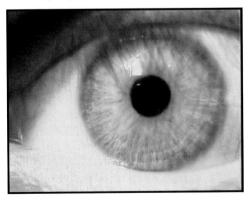

Physical Iris Description: a blue-to-blue gray iris with the appearance of loose wavy fibers. Aberrant fibers are often seen as well as a milky white area around the ruff zone. Pupil is sometimes enlarged and can be deformed. Nerve rings indicating stress and sensitivity of the nervous system are often found, usually in the outer rings of the iris.

General Complaints:

– General sensitivity to stress and tendency toward exhaustion caused by over-excitement.
– Sensitivity to weather changes and phases of the moon
– Weakness of the nerves
– Anxiety is common and many suffer from neuroses or variable moods

- Difficulty in overcoming emotional traumas
- Often these people are light sleepers
- May have migraine headaches, or dizziness as the nervous system affects circulation
- Congestion and inflammation of the lymphatic system
- Excessive mucus with a tendency to allergies
- Nervous stress can result in skin conditions, asthma, and nervous stomach or irritable bowel syndromes
- A fast pulse (tachycardia) is common
- Poor utilization of foods due to potent nervous influences

Common Complaints in Childhood:

- Fear, anxiety and high emotional sensitivity
- Very excitable, these types often eat and drink too fast which can result in burping and nervous vomiting
- Very sensitive to changes in the environment

Common Complaints in Adulthood:

- Easily hurt in relationships and highly sensitive
- Often have neuroses and may suffer from nervous breakdown if under a lot of stress
- Often worry unnecessarily over other people's problems
- Due to an overactive nervous system and a poor ability to utilize the B-group vitamins they require B-group vitamins in greater amounts
- Deficiencies in calcium, magnesium, and iron and zinc are commonly seen
- After the fifth decade, there is a tendency to develop muscle weakness, edema, and diabetes
- Nervous stomach, ulcers, and bowel problems
- Headaches or migraines
- Weakening of the adrenal glands
- In women, a disposition to cancer of the female organs

Hydro-lymphatic

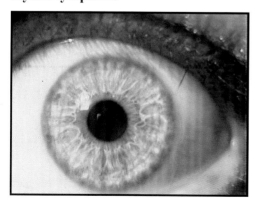

Physical Iris Description: a blue-to-blue gray iris, which may occasionally be brown with a blurred ring of clouds around the ruff zone as well as another ring of well-defined clouds in the outer ring of the iris. Clouds are often white but may be yellow, orange, or brown depending on degree of toxicity. In the brown eye there are larger clouds and the inner ring and outer ring of clouds are often joined together.

General Complaints:

- Chronic lymphatic congestion often with persistent infections
- Commonly suffer from asthma, bronchitis, colds and flu
- There are often weaknesses in the heart with high blood pressure or fluctuations in blood pressure
- Predisposition to rheumatoid arthritis
- Depression, mood changes, and impatience are often seen
- Perspire heavily but suffer from heavy fluid retention which can cause edema and weight fluctuations
- Predisposition to diseases of the urinary tract, urinary infections, gallstone and kidney stone formation and varicose veins
- Often there is minimal endurance

Common Complaints in Childhood:

- Recurrent bronchitis, colds, and flu
- Lymphatic congestion and low immunity to infections
- Prone to allergies

Common Complaints in Adulthood:

- Adults tend to develop a stocky physique with a large abdomen
- Due to fluid problems and edema, they may wake in the morning with a puffy face and eyelids that are swollen
- Cold and damp weather generally worsens their health problems
- Blue-eyed types are more prone to catarrhal problems with heavy mucus secretion like asthma and bronchitis, as well as heart weakness with high blood pressure
- Brown-eyed types often suffer from rheumatic problems and angina pectoris

Hematogenic

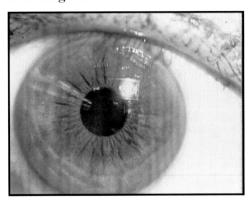

Physical Iris Description: a brown iris with a velvet sponge-like plaque over the eye. Nerve rings in the iris are commonly seen and radii solaris (deep channels from the pupil outwards).

General Features/Complaints:

- Often have olive colored skin and dark hair and stem from physically strong genetic backgrounds (Mediterranean, Asian, African)

- Cultural change in diet and lifestyle can greatly influence health in a negative way
- May display impulsive or hyperactive behavior and have a tendency to be over emotional and easily excited
- The overactive nervous system often causes problems for the heart and circulation, liver and gall bladder
- A rapid circulation, viscous blood and strong pulse often leads to varicose veins
- Asthma is common as well as problems with the thyroid gland

Common Complaints in Childhood:

- May be hyperactive and have difficulty in concentration
- Nervous stomach or cramps may occur
- Skin problems like eczema are likely
- Asthma or other respiratory diseases may be seen

Common Complaints in Adulthood:

- May loose temper easily or be over-emotional
- Digestive problems include slow moving bowels that can result in constipation, hemorrhoids and general toxicity, nervous stomach, dyspepsia or excessive intestinal gas
- Gallstones and kidney stones may form due to high levels of nitrogenous waste and uric acid in the blood
- Skin diseases are often found that develop into boils due to poor liver function
- After the age of 30 there is an greater chance of high cholesterol and angina pectoris
- Arteriosclerosis is often seen in later years as well as memory loss and reduced blood flow to the brain
- Varicose veins

Mixed Constitution

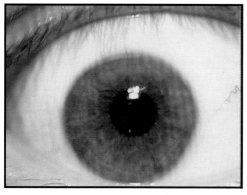

Physical Iris Description: a mixed blue and brown iris with brown pigment overlaid onto a base of blue fibers. Commonly there is a central brown pigment, which is the darkest area in the iris.

General Complaints:

- Gastrointestinal problems such as constipation and excessive intestinal gas

- Pancreatic problems in secretion of enzymes and control of blood sugar levels
- Liver and gallbladder complaints which can include problems in bile production and secretion
- Sensitive nervous system

Common Complaints in Childhood and Adulthood:

- Liver problems
- Constipation and/or diarrhea
- Nervous stomach or irritable bowel syndrome
- Flatulence
- Gallstones or gallbladder conditions
- Fluctuating blood sugar levels
- Reduction in digestive enzymes
- Dry skin or acne
- Frequent feelings of nausea
- Nerve weakness

Plethoric

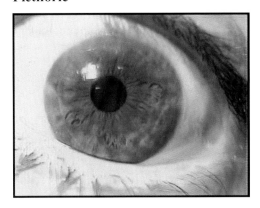

Physical Iris Description: a blue or brown iris with a generally small pupil and a rough- textured large ruff zone around the pupil, which usually bulges downward.

General Complaints:

- The term "plethora" means an excess amount of blood leading to a slowing down in movement which in this case relates to a sluggish venous flow of blood towards the heart
- Both adults and children are prone to become overweight
- Due to excessive blood in the skin, the complexion is often quite red and acne and skin complaints are frequent
- Disturbances in bile flow due to liver congestion which affects digestion
- Excessive production of mucus which can bring on asthma
- May exhibit variable moody or irritable behavior with depression
- Sleepiness, fatigue

Common Complaints in Childhood:

- Children of this type are often overweight
- Complexion is red and various skin problems or acne may develop
- Moodiness
- Colds, and sinus problems, and asthma is common

Common Complaints in Adulthood:

- Conditions of blood stagnation and congestion lead to problems like varicose veins, loss of tone in the veins, hemorrhoids and thromboses
- Frequent backaches often due to a blocked congested blood flow and extra weight gain in the abdomen area
- In later years angina pectoris is frequent
- Endocrine weakness especially in the thyroid gland
- High blood cholesterol and arteriosclerosis
- Liver problems with disturbances in bile flow
- Problems in digestion

Hormonal

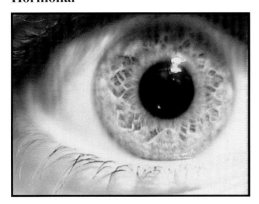

Physical Iris Description: a blue or brown iris with many lacunae or holes connected to the outside of the ruff zone. There are two types; the glandular type, which exhibits many evenly, sized lacunae and the pleuri-glandular type, which has larger and more varied lacunae.

General Complaints:

- The glandular type experiences functional hormonal problems while the pleuri-glandular suffers mainly from congenital degeneration of the glands
- The pleuri-glandular type is plagued by genetic problems and is harder to treat
- Hormonal disturbances including the pituitary, thyroid, parathyroid, adrenal, gonads, and pancreas
- Fluctuations in blood sugar and disturbances in mineral economy
- Possible disturbances in basal metabolism and thermo-regulation

Common Complaints in Childhood:

- Disturbance in the growth of bones which includes diseases like rickets
- Frequent inflammation of the tonsils and appendix

– May have growing pains as there tends to be an over production of some of the growth hormones and an accelerated rate of growth
– Teenage girls often have problems during menstruation and malfunction of the thyroid gland
– Tendency to develop puppy fat at an early age

Common Complaints in Adulthood:
– Symptoms are often minor until after the age of 50
– In women there may be irregular or painful menstruation and premature menopause
– In men the adrenal gland suffers leading to blood sugar fluctuations as well as prostate gland and circulation problems in later years
– Weakened pituitary, thyroid, adrenal and pancreas glands
– Thyroid gland problems contribute to fluctuations in body weight and metabolism and weakened hair growth
– Blood pressure fluctuations and dizziness are often complaints after the age of 35
– Fatigue, depression, lack of drive and a greater need for quality sleep
– Constipation and poor digestion
– In old age there is a tendency to develop cancer of the endocrine organs such as the uterus and prostate

Connective Tissue

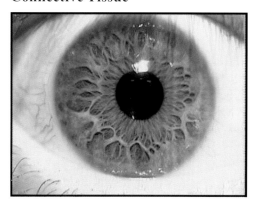

Physical Iris Description: a blue or brown iris with many large open and closed lacunae often reaching to the outer edge of the iris giving the eye a very dramatic look. There are several weakened areas in the fibers, which create a loose structure and very weak fiber density.

General Complaints:
– Connective tissue weakness which often involves the prolapsing or dropping of organs especially in the abdomen
– Weak connective tissues and ligaments may create pain in the long bones and joints of the body as well as frequent injuries to ankles
– Poor and slow recovery and healing of injuries due to a weak immune system
– Insufficient energy and oxygen metabolism leading to poor endurance, constant fatigue and frequent shortness of breath
– Problems generally improve in a warmer climate

- Accumulation of waste products in kidneys and connective tissue creating irritation of muscles and connective tissue and arthritic problems
- Poor posture, weak bones and spinal problems are common
- Weakness in the metabolism of Vitamin C and bioflavonoids
- Connective tissue weakness also affects the bowel, glands, nerves, heart, and circulation

Common Complaints in Childhood:

- Children have thin, loose skin giving them the appearance of being older than their age
- Often there is overstretching of the joints

Common Complaints in Adulthood:

- Hemorrhoids, varicose veins, and hernias
- Weak bones and spinal problems like scoliosis
- Feel tired easily
- Loss of tone and elasticity of the blood vessels leading to circulation problems
- Women often have menstrual problems, abdominal and pelvic difficulties, and infertility due to mild prolapse of the uterus and pelvic organs, which can also put pressure on the bladder and cause irritation
- In older age there may be heart complaints and the face is often heavily wrinkled with loose, hanging skin
- Knee and ankle joint problems
- Organs prolapse especially abdominal

Chapter 3
The iris of the eye at first glance

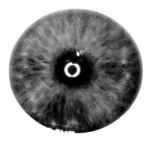

"The iridologist must take a deeper look and learn the language of the iris."

To adequately understand how accurate analysis is made through iridology, it is important to take a look at the iris and its appearance. We have previously seen that there exist several genetic iris constitutions, each with different characteristics. However, every person is an individual and while knowledge of the patient's genetic type is greatly helpful, we must look further to discover the entire picture of the individual's weaknesses.

The iris of the eye can be divided into several zones. As shown below, these consist of the pupil, pupil border, ruff zone, ruff border, ciliary zone, lymphatic and blood zone, skin zone, and the sclera, or the white of the eye. Each of these zones will now be described in greater detail.

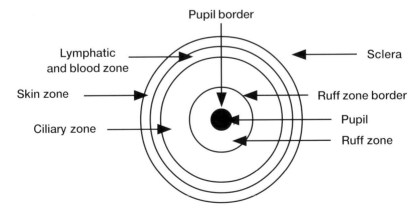

At the center of the iris lie the pupil and the pupil border which, as we will learn in later chapters reveal conditions of the spine, nervous system and a number of psychological indicators of health status. The "ruff zone" named because of the high shirt collars or ruffs that used to be worn, encircles the pupil. Its size, shape, color and texture, reveal the status of the digestive system, an area of great importance to be investigated in a later chapter.

The ruff border represents our autonomic nervous system. Within the ciliary zone, lie all our organs, some of which include the kidneys, liver, heart, brain, lungs, glands, as well as others. It is this zone, in which the thousands of signs and marks are usually displayed, and which is the language the iris uses to reflect the status of our organs. The next ring around the iris reveals the lymphatic and blood circulation while skin condition is shown in the outermost ring. One must not forget the sclera, or the white of the eye because within it we often find colors, flecks, and several types of veins that indicate other potential problems.

The competent iridologist will examine each of these zones very carefully and by using this information along with an understanding of the patient's genetic constitution, can make a more accurate diagnosis.

It is very important to stress that iridology allows one to examine the entire health status of an individual. It is a mistake to take into account only a mark or a spot in a specific organ area and conclude for example that the patient has a weak liver. My years in iridology have taught me to look at a variety of signs to confirm a diagnosis. The experienced iridologist should have knowledge of physiology and anatomy and should examine the entire iris, as all the organs in the body are interrelated and dependent on each other. This is called the "holistic approach" the one that modern medicine often forgets.

What tools does an iridologist use to perform an iris diagnosis?

Up to recent times, the analysis of the iris had been made using magnifying lenses. This method is still being used today, but I find this method quite limited as only a superficial diagnosis can be made this way. This aside, it is usually quite uncomfortable for the patients who must keep their eyes wide open while the iridologist examines the iris, reducing the time and accuracy of the iris diagnosis. A professional iridologist should use a system of analysis that captures an image or photograph of the iris using a microscope camera. Modern computer technology now allows manipulation of captured iris images so that, for example, dark brown eyes, which were previously difficult to analyze, can with the aid of computer technology reveal the necessary iris structures to enable a thorough analysis.

The iridologist also uses an iris map or chart to assist in locating specific organ areas. A variety of maps have been developed around the world but from my study of several thousand irises, I have developed my own iris chart, which is described in more detail in chapter five.

Chapter 4

Treat the Cause not only the symptoms of disease

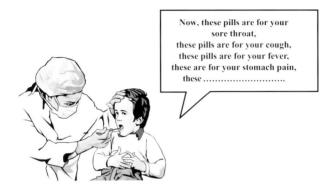

"The root of the problem is often masked by many symptoms."

There once lived two men who each had a wooden pail of water to drink that would hang from one of the branches of a tree in their yards. One day, they both found that their water pail had begun to leak.

The first man would add some extra water every day so that his pail of water stayed full. After several days he became tired of filling the pail every day and decided to use some glue to fix the hole. The pail of water once again stayed full but after a week, it began to leak again. The man found that there was another leak and again took the glue and fixed the second leak. And so it went on week after week, as he filled each additional hole with glue. He was satisfied with this system as it saved him time filling the pail every day. All he had to worry about every week was repairing just another new hole.

The second man, who discovered that his pail of water was leaking, asked himself "Why is my pail leaking?" He found a small hole at the bottom of the pail, and then asked, " Why is this hole in the pail?" He discovered that a woodpecker that lived in the tree made the hole in the pail. He fixed the hole with some glue, hung the pail on his fence instead, and never had a leak again.

One major area of confusion that needs to be explained is that iridology generally reveals mainly the status of the organs and systems in the body, it does not usually reveal a disease, although in some cases it may be possible. Many a patient had unnecessarily been disappointed that his iridologist did not identify in the iris diagnosis a specific disease from which he suffered. I have an explanation for this behavior. We have been taught to cure the disease and not the cause of the disease. Over the last 200 years or so, modern medicine has created names for every possible disease known to exist. Many of these diseases have no cure but they have a name. I have often spoken to patients who had been through a variety of classical examinations and clinical tests where no disease was found, yet they have symptoms that reveal a problem and it had shown up in their irises. In some cases, my patients have come to me in dire need because no diagnosis of a problem had been made and their doctors attributed their symptoms to psychological causes and recommended a visit to the psychiatrist!

It is nice to know the name of a disease in modern medicine since there is usually a nice chemical drug that can treat it, but are we treating the cause of the disease or just the symptoms? If we are not using a holistic approach, we are not really treating the whole person's problems. To do this, we must look for the cause of the disease or the root of the problem and that is where iris diagnosis shows great advantage. If we believe that the body is composed of interconnected systems, each of those systems is composed of interconnected organs, and each of those organs is composed of interconnected cells, then we have to believe that if the cells of each organ receive what they require every day, we can build a strong, well-balanced body that will resist any infection or disease that may attack it. Obviously, we must also take into account our environment, diet, genetics, and stress in our lives that change the demands on the cells of our bodies and we must compensate for this to stay healthy.

If you understand these principles then you will understand why I believe that iris diagnosis is the greatest method we have for locating the causes of our health problems providing a complete holistic approach to discovering the cause of disease, and not just a superficial, candy-coated treatment to make the symptoms go away.

May your pail of water always be full!

Chapter 5

The eyes are maps to our bodies

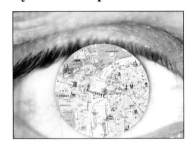

"A map is only a guide to see the whole picture. There are countless ways to reach our destination but without a map we are often lost. We use our intuition, our feelings, our heart, our knowledge from past experience, and our brain and logic to determine which path we must take.
Use these tools of life to discover a new world, one that will lead you to your chosen destiny"

What is an Iris Map?

In Chapter 3 we learned how an iridologist examines the iris of the eye and that it is composed of several zones representing different segments of the body. We learned that one of the tools an iridologist uses is an iris map.

An iris map or chart is a graphical representation of where specific body organs or systems are located in the iris of the human eye. These maps identify not only the iris zones, but any structures that may be found within each of these zones. Iris maps have been developed through studies of thousands and thousands of patients who have had the same specific problems in various areas of the body. Ignatz von Peczely discovered that patients who had the same medical problem had similar signs in the same location of the iris. Over the last one hundred years, the iris has been studied and mapped and today relatively accurate maps allow the iridologist to locate the specific body organs that are reflected in the iris of the eye.

It should be noted that iris maps only provide the iridologist with a guide. Through my experience, I have come to the realistic conclusion that no single patient will have for example, a certain body organ in the same exact location as the iris maps depict; each of us is unique. There may be a slight variation in its location, within certain limits.

Use the iris map to get a general understanding of where body organs lie in the iris but as variations do occur, be careful not to take it as gospel truth, or you may fail to make an accurate analysis. As we will see in future chapters, there are many other signs that can be located in the iris to confirm your initial diagnosis. The iris map however, provides an excellent way to view the individual health status of the whole body and to see how each body organ and system is dependent on each other.

History of Iris Maps

Although the history of iridology as we learned in the first chapter, dates back hundreds of years, Ignatz von Peczely developed the first iris map in the year 1886, the same bright individual who discovered the changes in the eyes of an owl. For the first time in history, a graphical representation of what is seen in the iris was published for the world to see. This was to change the face of iridology forever and form a base of knowledge that would be expanded upon by the many great iridologists who were to follow. Even though this initial map indicated only the basic structures, many of the organs that we associate with specific areas of the iris have remained in the same location on the iris maps since this first map was designed over 100 years ago. Renowned European iridologists such as Nils Liljequist, Josef Angerer, Josef Deck and American iridologists Henry Edward Lane, Henry Lindlahr, and Bernard Jensen, later developed iris maps.

It is interesting that all these maps developed in different parts of the world are up to about 85 percent in agreement with each other, even though many were designed without prior knowledge of the existence of any other maps. I believe, that with the ever-advancing computer technology our knowledge of iridology will rapidly expand and thus, in future years, we may be able to gain even more information about the human body from more accurate mapping of the iris to help us in reaching even more exact diagnoses.

Like the early pioneers and explorers who developed maps for us to see the world as we know it, iridologists search for a greater understanding of the iris terrain which measures a little less than a small coin. There is still so much to know and understand about the language of the iris just as there is to understand about the depths of the oceans or the great-unknown expanse of space around us. We human beings have come up with thousands of inventions, built enormous machines, buildings and structures. We have designed many electronic methods and diagnostic machines, which attempt to uncover only a fraction of what may possibly exist. Man has designed machines and as we often see, these machines are not perfect and subject to error. The iris of the eye cannot lie or make a mistake, only we as iridologists can misinterpret what it is telling us.

The iris map that I have designed through studies of thousands of patients is explained and described below. Let it guide you through the magnificent terrain we call the human iris and reveal some of the mysteries of the human body that have always amazed me, as well as countless iridologists, over the past one hundred years.

Explanation of the Iris Map

The iris map describes the right and left iris with the iris divided into segments of a clock. Between each of the time zones, lie general body zones, including the brain, face, mouth and throat, spine, kidney-sexual, lower and upper abdominal, respiratory-heart, and shoulder-neck zones. These zones are also depicted by drawings of their major organs, which encircle the iris map.

Frank Navratil, BSc. N. D.

IRIDOLOGY CHART
ACCORDING TO
FRANK NAVRATIL BSc. N. D.
© copyright 2000

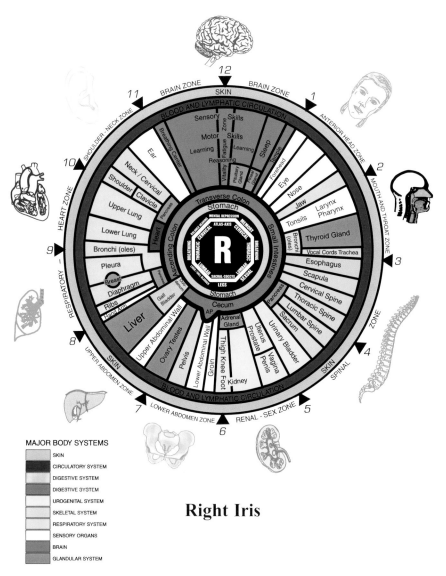

Right Iris

MAJOR BODY SYSTEMS

- SKIN
- CIRCULATORY SYSTEM
- DIGESTIVE SYSTEM
- DIGESTIVE SYSTEM
- UROGENITAL SYSTEM
- SKELETAL SYSTEM
- RESPIRATORY SYSTEM
- SENSORY ORGANS
- BRAIN
- GLANDULAR SYSTEM

IRIDOLOGY CHART
ACCORDING TO
FRANK NAVRATIL BSc. N. D.
© copyright 2000

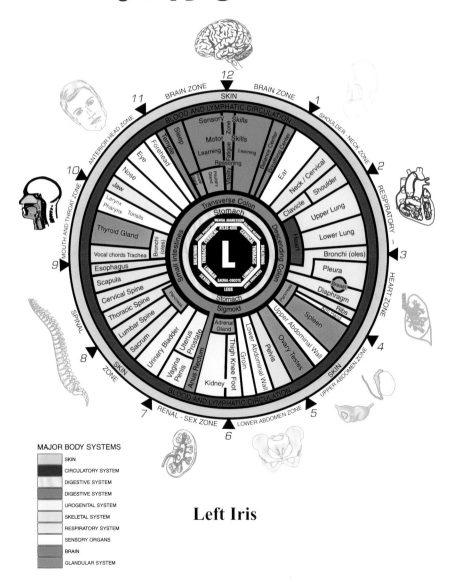

Left Iris

MAJOR BODY SYSTEMS

- SKIN
- CIRCULATORY SYSTEM
- DIGESTIVE SYSTEM
- DIGESTIVE SYSTEM
- UROGENITAL SYSTEM
- SKELETAL SYSTEM
- RESPIRATORY SYSTEM
- SENSORY ORGANS
- BRAIN
- GLANDULAR SYSTEM

Organs that lie on the left side of the body can be seen in the left iris map, while organs that lie on the right side of the body are seen in the right iris map. Paired organs such as the lungs and kidneys as well as the organs that lie in the middle of the body, such as the intestines, brain, and spine can be seen in both irises. Generally, the top of the body is seen in the top part of the iris map while lower organs are located in the lower regions of the map.

The main body systems are color coded for easier identification. These include the skin, circulatory, digestive, urogenital, skeletal, respiratory, sensory organ, brain, and endocrine systems.

Starting from the center we see the black pupil. An octagon has been drawn inside the pupil to describe the various types of pupil flattening that occur and what implications they have on the physical and psychological health status of the individual. Pupil flattening will be dealt with specifically in much greater detail in the chapter, "The Pupil."

Surrounding the pupil is the "ruff zone", where the digestive system is located. The light brown area reflects the stomach ring and the darker brown area reveals the small and large intestines and appendix. Other organs related to digestion and shown in brown color are the duodenum, gall bladder, anus and rectum, and esophagus. Signs seen in these areas will be revealed in the "Digestive System" chapter.

As we move outwards from the digestive system, we find the ciliary zone which houses the many organs of the body.

The respiratory system shown in blue includes the vocal chords, pleura, diaphragm, lungs, bronchi, bronchioles, and trachea.

The circulatory system is shown in red and consists of the left heart in the left iris and the right heart in the right iris as well as the blood and lymphatic circulation, located in the outer ring of the iris map.

The urogenital system is shown in yellow color and includes the kidney, urinary bladder, prostate gland, uterus, vagina, and penis.

The skeletal system in green reveals the segments of the spinal column as well as the neck, jaw, shoulder, clavicle, scapula, pelvis, and ribs.

The sensory organs including the eyes, nose and ears are depicted in light blue.

The brain, in purple color is shown between 11 and 1 o'clock in the upper portion of the iris.

The endocrine system consisting of the pituitary, pineal, thyroid, pancreas, adrenal glands as well as the spleen, breast, ovaries, testes and liver are located in various regions of the ciliary zone in orange color.

The tonsils, larynx, pharynx, forehead, hand and arm, groin, and upper and lower abdominal walls are pictured in white.

Finally the outermost ring in pink is the skin zone.

Have a closer look at the iris map and become familiar with where the body organs lie. This will provide a base of understanding for the chapters that follow.

Chapter 6

Eye Colors

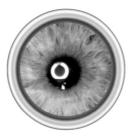

"We have always been aware of the color of people's eyes but do we know what makes these colors the way they are?"

Since ancient times man has always been fascinated with the color of eyes. Often when asked what physical features one looks at when choosing a partner, eye color is mentioned. What is it about the color of our eyes that we find so captivating? We use our eyes to communicate our feelings, and emotions. Often our eyes describe our character and words like powerful, hypnotizing, gentle, kind, sad, and angry come to mind in their description.

Our eyes have always been the center of attention. People notice right away if the person they are talking to does not look them in the eye. Often this behavior denotes that one is shy or is not telling the truth and cannot be trusted. There is a great deal of information about one another that we interpret from our eyes.

How many eye colors are there? Let's take a brief count; blue, green, brown, black, light brown, dark brown, hazel green, gray, light blue, dark blue, yellow green, blue gray, turquoise, and the thousands of shades in between. We use eye color to identify people or criminals but do we really know why there are so many different eye colors? From studying irises and eye colors for many years, I have come to the conclusion that there exist only 2 true eye colors, brown and blue. This belief is also shared by a number of iridologists around the world. They believe that dating back thousands of years, the blue-eyed races migrated to the cooler climates such as Northern Europe and the brown-eyed races migrated to the warmer climates like Africa.

Blue irises are often associated with fair skin and blonde hair but there are blue-eyed people with dark skin and dark hair. There are some general tendencies of blue-eyed types to have predispositions to tonsillitis, swollen lymphatic glands, respiratory problems, and acne or eczema and arthritic or rheumatic problems in old age.

Brown irises are often associated with dark skin and dark hair although the opposite can also occur. Tendencies for brown-eyed people are to develop problems with the liver and circulation, hemorrhoids and thromboses, diabetes, digestive problems, and disturbances of the hormonal system.

Due to interracial mixing over thousands of years, we now have the mixture of colors that we presently see.

However, how do we explain changes in eye color during one's life? My extensive iris studies have consistently demonstrated that eye color can and does change due to changes in health status throughout life. This occurrence even dates back to Ignatz von Peczely who first noticed that changes in color from black to white occurred in the eyes of an owl. What many do not realize is, that if you take a close look at the human iris it is generally not just one color.

Within the iris are often seen clouds and flecks and a variety of different marks in several different colors that change during one's life.

If we take into account that genetics play a role in eye color, which, as we have seen in the number of genetic iris constitutions as true, we must also take into account changes in eye color during the life of the individual. We are born with an iris constitution that generally stays with us our entire lives. This is not to say that slight changes in constitution do not occur because I believe, that in a hundred years we will have a whole new set of genetic constitutions, each with different physical and psychological characteristics. Perhaps due to the increasing amount of interracial mixing, fewer and fewer genetic types will be seen. Maybe in the future there will be only one genetic type, meaning that every person will have the same make-up and the same mixture of colors in the eye. This is only a speculation but food for thought!

If we ignore the eye color that is due to our genetic make-up we are left with colors in the eye that are there because of changes that occur in our bodies. I believe along with thousands of iridologists around the world, that these colors represent changes in our physical health status.

Let's take a look at the colors and pigments that are found in the iris of the eye and what they mean in iridology.

Brown

Brown color pigment can be found in blue or brown eyes. There are a variety of shades of this pigment but all refer to changes in liver function.

If the brown pigment is found in the ruff zone, it is often indicative of inadequate and low quality bile production, which will affect the digestion of fats and lead to conditions like constipation and nausea.

If the brown pigment is found in the ciliary zone, it could have been acquired or inherited, but no matter where it is found, it indicates secondary liver problems. In liver cirrhosis due to alcohol, there are often a number of brown flecks throughout both of the irises indicating the vast extent of functions that the liver has in our body.

If the iris has a brown haze over it, it could reveal degeneration of the liver creating general toxicity in the blood and tissues. More information about liver signs will be given in a future chapter.

Patients are often alarmed when they discover dark brown flecks in their eyes, but many may have had them since birth. This is not to say that they do not mean anything.

They may have inherited weaknesses in the liver from their parents or even during birth due to certain drugs. I have often seen brown flecks appear after certain medications had been taken, or after a high use of drugs, again indicating liver damage. These flecks may lighten with healthy living but will not usually disappear completely.

Orange

Orange color can be found in both brown or blue eye types although it may be more difficult to see in brown eyes without computer technology. The orange pigment can be bright orange or orange-brown. Generally, when this pigment is seen one or both functions of the pancreas may be weakened; the exocrine function (secretion of digestive enzymes) and the endocrine function (regulation of blood sugar and insulin).

If the orange pigment is found in the ruff zone it is usually in flecks and may indicate that the production of pancreatic enzymes is lacking at times.

If the orange-brown pigment is found there and covers a large part of the ruff zone, there may be a combination of reduced pancreatic enzymes together with inadequate or poor bile from the liver and gall bladder.

In the ciliary zone orange pigment is often found on or outside the ruff border and can indicate fluctuations in blood sugar. This pigment is sometimes seen as sprinklings of orange color. Low blood sugar levels may also be seen by orange color in the brain area affecting memory and concentration levels.

Yellow

Yellow pigment can be found in both blue and brown-eye types. In the brown eye it appears to make the brown a lighter color. When seen in the blue eye it will make the eye appear green at a distance. I have never seen a true green eye and after analyzing thousands, I am convinced that a green eye really has a basic blue structure with overlying yellow flecks. When this pigment is seen, the kidneys may be weakened or there may be problems with uric acid metabolism.

If the ruff zone contains yellow pigment, it may indicate diarrhea while in the ciliary zone it indicates depressed kidney function and problems with uric acid metabolism.

Red

Red pigment indicates problems in the hormonal system specifically the pituitary gland. This red pigment is occasionally seen along ridges that stem from the ruff zone out to the ciliary zone which are called radii solarii. Alternatively, there may be red or reddish-brown pigments throughout all or in any part of the iris.

Beige or orange-yellow mist

This color seen as a mist rather than distinct clouds is indicative of thyroid problems. Along with this color can be seen fluctuations in weight, fatigue, rapid or slowing heartbeat or heart palpitations, and fluid retention.

White

White color in the iris indicates acute inflammation of the indicated area.

If seen in the ruff zone it often indicates over-acidity of the stomach and/or the intestines.

Excessive white color generally indicates an over-acid condition of the body leading to problems like arthritis, and gout.

Gray

Gray color is generally seen in lacunae, where a hole has been formed in the iris and indicates a chronic or pre-chronic stage of tissue degeneration. At times, this gray color can be seen in the stomach zone, which may indicate degeneration or atrophy of the secretory cells of the stomach.

Black

One must be careful not to confuse black coloring with dark brown as black is a color that is quite rare to see in the iris of the eye.

Near black color or very dark gray indicates severe degeneration of the organ. Black color indicates tissue inactivity or tissue death where there is irreversible damage to that body organ. Black or near black can be seen in some cancer conditions.

Other colors

There are sometimes other colors occasionally seen in the iris. Many are due to mixtures of the colors mentioned above. Some drugs can also create unusual colors appearing in the iris. Violet color can sometimes appear in the ruff zone indicating a predisposition to diabetes.

Genetic colors

Occasionally, a person may be born with one blue and one brown eye, one eye half brown and half blue, or a mixture of blue and brown as in the mixed constitution mentioned in an earlier chapter.

Eye color throughout one's life generally changes due to the body degenerating and becoming more toxic and this is often attributed to inappropriate nutrition, accumulation of drugs taken, genetic make-up, sedentary lifestyle, and stress.

With natural therapies like mega dose vitamin therapy and improved nutrition and lifestyle changes, I have seen positive changes in eye color occur. This means that some of the toxic colors that appear can slowly disappear or become less noticeable. For some individuals these positive changes can take up to 5 years, depending on the toxicity and degeneration present. There have been cases where an iris that appeared to be brown began to slowly change to blue with natural therapy, indicating that there had been a severe toxic condition in the body.

Eye color is a very important and useful indicator in iridology. It assists the iridologist in locating and focusing on general problem conditions in the body.

(Examples of iris colors)

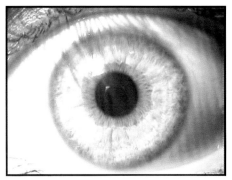

Yellow

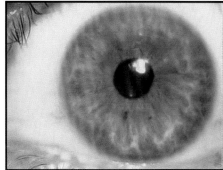

Orange

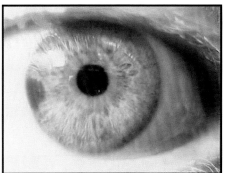

Brown

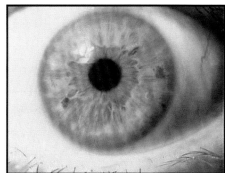

Misty beige

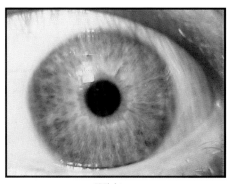

White

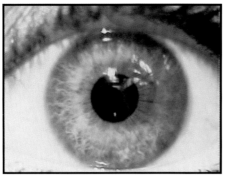 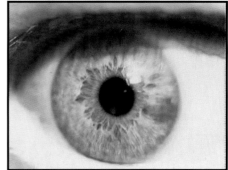

Genetic colors   Genetic colors

Chapter 7

Fundamental Iris Signs

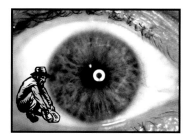

"The iridologist is like a pioneer uncovering the secrets of the hidden landscape of the iris terrain."

We have seen that the language of the iris reveals colors that indicate potential or existing problems in the body. We have also seen how our genetic make-up is revealed through genetic iris constitutions each with its own set of physical and sometimes psychological characteristics.

Once we gain an appreciation of the genetic iris constitution and the colors that exist in the iris, we can begin to probe deeper into the fascinating landscape of the iris terrain. We will discover that the iris surface is not a smooth surface but on closer inspection, is composed of hills, valleys and depressions much like the surface of the earth or the moon.

Listed below are some of the most often seen general signs and markings in the iris and what each of them means in iridology. Iridologists have discovered many over the last one hundred years. Specific signs that relate to certain organs or conditions will be revealed in their respective chapters. Remember that marks in the iris do not indicate damage to the iris or the eye itself but reflect conditions that are present in the body. It should also be stressed that iris signs cannot usually reveal that the patient has undergone an operation where there has been removal of body organs like the gall bladder or female organs. Some believe that while under anesthesia, the nervous system is blocked and signs are not recorded in the iris during that time. The same goes for gallstones or kidney stones since they have no nerve supply. Therefore, their presence is not recorded in the iris. Pregnancy is a natural state and not a disease state so it cannot be seen as a sign in the iris.

The following list is by no means a complete list of iris signs, as thousands have been discovered and debated on over the past century, and I am sure more will be uncovered in the future. The signs and markings that are included are those that I have seen most often through my personal iris studies.

A. Lacunae

Lacunae are breaks that occur in the fibers of the iris and form an oval shape which can be open (open lacuna), or closed (closed lacuna). Other common shapes include ellipse-shaped (ellipsoid lacuna), needle-shaped (needle lacuna), the shape of a bird's beak (bird's beak lacuna), leaf shaped (leaf lacuna), asparagus tip shaped (asparagus tip lacuna) or hole-shaped (hole lacuna).

They all indicate areas of weakness in the location where they are found. Their degree of weakness is determined by the type of lacuna as well as the level of tissue change (explained in a later chapter).

1. Open Lacuna

An open lacuna is a lesion that is open at one or both ends.

This type of lacunae indicates a lowered activity of the organ but metabolic processes are still in operation. They can be found in any area of the iris but are frequently seen in the kidney, heart or thyroid areas. This condition is easier to heal but if left untreated can degenerate to a closed lacuna.

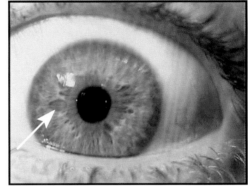

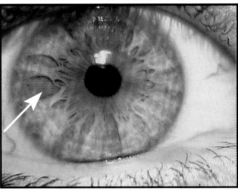

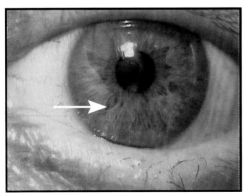

2. Closed Lacuna

A closed lacuna is a lesion that is oval in shape and totally encircled. When seen in the iris, it indicates a more severe form of tissue weakness and often there is restricted blood and nerve supply with toxins that cannot be eliminated. It represents a process that has come to an end and healing is harder to achieve than with the open lacuna. Small black closed lacunae can indicate tumor formation.

3. Ellipsoid lacuna

An ellipsoid lacuna is a closed lacuna in the shape of an ellipse. It is usually found in the glandular areas near the ruff zone. It indicates a pre-disposition to a cancerous condition. When seen pushing up the ruff border, it may be a sign of possible neoplasm.

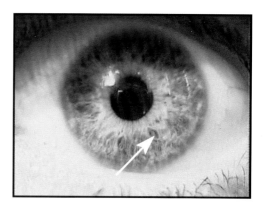

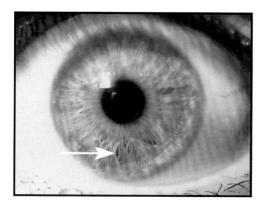

4. Needle lacuna

A needle lacuna is a very small, dark thin lacuna with both of its ends pointed. This type of lacuna indicates a high chance of degeneration, often leading to malignancy in the tissue or organ where it is found. Often there are signs of activity around this lacuna including white inflammation signs or bright markings, indicating an active condition.

5. Bird's beak lacuna

A bird's beak lacuna is a closed lacuna with one end pointed and the other rounded like the shape of a bird's beak. These lacunae are usually found outside the ruff border and indicate problems with the thyroid gland.

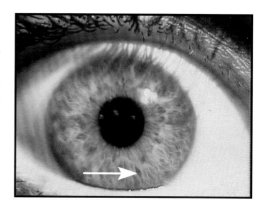

6. Leaf lacuna

A leaf lacuna is a closed lacuna with fibers running inside of it that gives it the appearance of a leaf. This sign often reveals a general hormonal imbalance and problems with the endocrine glands.

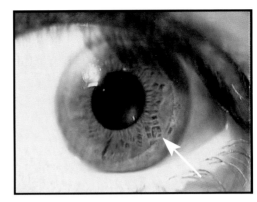

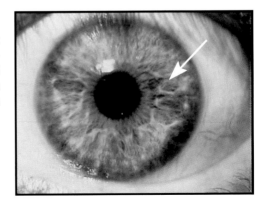

7. Asparagus tip lacuna

The asparagus tip lacuna begins near the ruff border and extends out into the ciliary zone where it forms a wider tip, resembling the tip of an asparagus. When this sign is seen it indicates a potential chance of developing a tumor in the testes, ovaries, or the pituitary gland.

8. Hole Lacuna

The hole lacuna is a very small, dark gray to black break in the fibers resembling a small hole. It can be found anywhere in the iris and may indicate extensive degeneration leading to the formation of ulcers or cysts.

B. Transversals

Transversals are white fibers that run against the natural grain of iris fibers.

They may be found in any area of the iris including the ruff zone. Occasionally they are red and vascular which indicates a serious condition that requires urgent attention as blood congestion and poor circulation may lead to a rapid worsening of the present condition.

Often transversals are indicative of adhesions after operations, congestion in blood flow through organs where they are found, inflammation, or imbalance in the nervous system. A number of specific types can be found.

1. Spleen - Heart transversal

This transversal appears only in the left eye and starts from the spleen area up towards the heart. Usually it is vascular and may indicate decreased circulation to the heart muscle leading to angina pectoris or heart attack. It is not seen very often but when seen it denotes a grave condition.

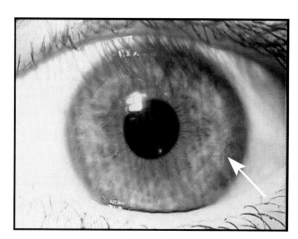

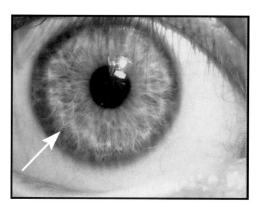

2. Liver -Gall Bladder transversal

This transversal is sometimes seen in the liver or gall bladder area, indicating inflammation of the gall bladder or liver, and if vascular, congestion of blood flow through the liver which can place a strain on the right chamber of the heart.

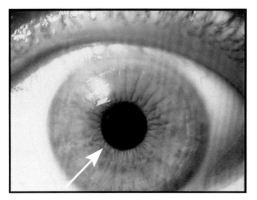

3. Digestive transversal

This transversal is seen in the ruff zone or digestive area and often indicates a nervous stomach or reduced or blocked enervation to the intestines, which may affect peristalsis, and create conditions like constipation, or diarrhea.

C. Lymphatic Clouds

Lymphatic clouds are found in the blood and lymphatic circulation zone in the form of a rosary of small beads or clouds that encircle part or the entire iris. They usually indicate

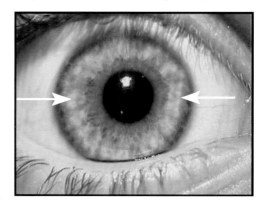

a poorly functioning lymphatic system prone to swollen or blocked lymphatic glands. This is often due to improperly digested fats that reduce the effectiveness of the lymphatic system and compromise the immune system. When these clouds turn yellow or brown they indicate a more chronic condition.

These clouds may sometimes shift closer inside the iris or form vertically. This is most often seen in the respiratory zone, which usually indicates congestion in the lungs or sometimes acute or chronic respiratory infections.

D. Arcus Senilus

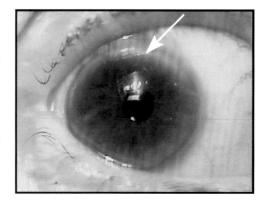

The Arcus Senilus sign is seen quite often especially in old age, although I have seen it in patients as young as 30 years old. It shows up in the top portion of the iris as a white arc. This sign indicates poor oxygenation to the brain and excessive buildup of cholesterol leading to arteriosclerosis or senility. It is the result of a lifetime of unhealthy living, poor nutrition and inactivity.

E. Cholesterol Ring

The cholesterol ring is similar to the Arcus Senilus but is found as a white ring around the iris other than just the top portion. This is also due to increased cholesterol and triglycerides in the blood, deposits of sodium or fatty material in arteries, which may lead to hardening of the arteries, calcium deposits, heart and/or joint problems.

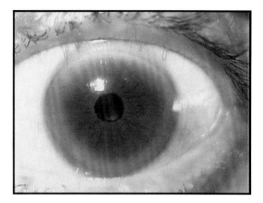

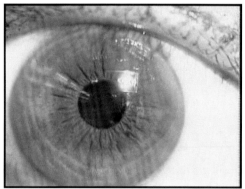

F. Nerve Rings

Nerve rings are channels that are seen running along the circumference of the iris, usually in the ciliary zone. They form as a result of cramping of the iris fibers due to nervous tension in the body. There may be one, two, three and even four rings indicating the degree of nervous tension. Breaks in the nerve ring can indicate restriction or inefficient functioning in the affected organs.

The color of the rings can also be an indicator as white nerve rings often reflect an irritation of the nervous system, while darker rings can indicate nerve damage. Nerve rings are most often seen in the Hematogenic and Neurolymphatic iris constitutions although they can occur in any types.

Chronic stress conditions are often the source of stress rings but I have even

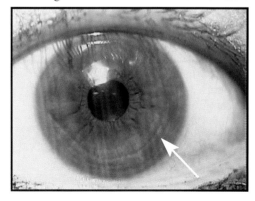

seen young children display stress rings in their irises. This may be due to inheriting nervous tension from their parents who live under stressful conditions or a stressful pregnancy where tension has been passed on to the child. Whatever the reason, it is always important when stress rings are seen, to allow the body and mind to relax for some time every day, to deal with negative emotions, and be at peace with yourself and your environment.

G. Radii Solarii

Radii Solarii are rays or channels that originate in the ruff zone and move outward to the ciliary zone. They are most often seen radiating upwards toward the brain area. This indicates a very toxic digestive system, which is beginning to affect organs where the sign travels. In the brain zone, toxicity here can affect the pituitary or pineal gland, or bring on headaches and migraines. If the radii solaris are observed in the lower regions of the iris, this can affect other hormonal glands such as the adrenal or pancreas. The deeper and darker they become, the greater the deposition of toxic materials in other organs of the body.

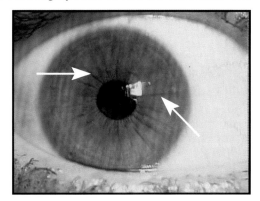

H. Darkening of the Ciliary Border

The outermost ring around the iris near the ciliary border is the skin zone. When a dark band occurs here, this indicates poor removal of toxins from the skin. The severity of the condition depends on how dark and wide the band is. Patients with this sign are more susceptible to skin problems.

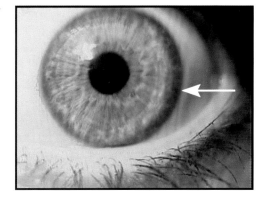

I. Iris Bulge

The Iris Bulge sign is seen when the iris exhibits an egg shape and one or both sides bulge outward. This sign indicates a reduced circulation to the head and a Vitamin B3 deficiency combined with problems with digestion. It is most often seen in the Neurolymphatic iris constitution due to their extra need for Vitamin B complex but it can also be seen in other types.

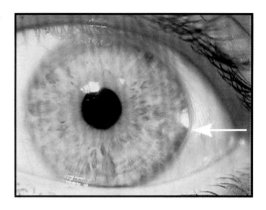

J. Ruff Border

The Ruff Border encircles the digestive or ruff zone. This represents the autonomic nervous system. If the border is white this indicates inflammation of the nerves. If there are breaks in the ruff border or if the border is poorly defined, this may reveal diminished nerve supply to organs that lie adjacent to where the break is located. It may also indicate intestinal insufficiency and a malabsorption of nutrients. More about the ruff border and ruff zone as it relates to the digestive system will be discussed in a later chapter.

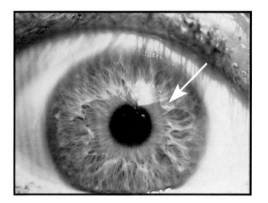

Chapter 8

The 5 stages of tissue change and the Healing Crisis

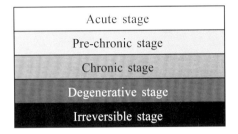

"You can fool yourself, but you can't fool your body—Have you really cured your disease?"

How can an iridologist determine how weak or how critical the patient's condition really is?

As mentioned earlier, when we look at the surface of the iris with a microscope we notice that it is not really smooth but full of ridges and valleys like the surface of the moon. There are various crevices and deeper areas in the ciliary zone that determine the shade of eye color. The deeper the ridges or crypts in the eye, the more the dark pigment epithelium shows through. The iris fibers that we see are actually formed of three or four layers of blood vessels coated with connective tissue and imbedded in the stroma.

Iridology reveals that the fibers running radially outward from the pupil are sometimes seen to lie above the surface of the iris and sometimes appear to sink to deeper levels. When the iris fibers lie above the surface of the iris, they appear lighter in color, white when in a blue iris and light yellow when seen in a brown iris. As the fibers sink to deeper levels, the color appears darker to become almost black in the deepest levels.

For iridologists this is a magnificent sign determining at what stage of tissue activity the patient's organs currently may be in.

In order to evaluate the condition of an organ in the body, I use a classification that places the level of tissue change into five distinct stages. These are: acute, pre-chronic, chronic, degenerative and irreversible. Each of these stages of tissue change will now be discussed in greater detail.

The **acute stage** is detected as an increase in the prominence of the superficial iris fibers. This makes them appear light in color and as mentioned, white in a blue iris and light yellow in a brown iris. This phenomenon is a result of inflammation in the particular organ represented by an increased blood supply and lymph to the area, which can result in pain, fever, or inflammation of tissue and discharge. The greater the acute activity, the greater is the change toward extreme acidity in body tissues. Whenever there is acidity there is catarrh, phlegm or mucus to carry the acids away to be eliminated. Acute conditions can result from vitamin and mineral deficiency, mechanical irritation, or bacterial invasion. Normally when a patient exhibits acute symptoms, modern medicine generally attempts to suppress the acute symptoms with a variety of suppressant drugs. Take the common cold, for example. Modern medicine is constantly searching for a cure for the common cold and today billions of dollars are spent on drugs that help us relieve conditions like sniffling, sneezing, runny nose, clogged sinuses etc.

Until this time though no scientist or medical expert has found a cure. But is the common cold really a disease? I believe the common cold is not a disease but a reaction that occurs as our bodies attempt to get rid of acidity by way of mucus and phlegm when the body is in an acute stage of inflammation. This implies that if we take suppressant drugs this will only push the problem to a deeper level. This in turn, only touches the surface of the problem because without proper diet and lifestyle habits, the root of the problem remains and the acute stage will retreat to the next stage of tissue change, the pre-chronic stage.

The **pre-chronic stage** appears in the iris of the eye as a grayish white or paler yellow as the iris fibers are not as elevated and appear to recede back into the stroma of the eye. This stage is represented by less blood and lymph and nerve activity to the associated organ and a lower metabolic rate. There is often less pain and discharge than at the acute stage, and often the patient believes that he is cured, when in fact, he is not. Again if proper nutrition and lifestyle habits are not corrected, the patient will regress to the next level of tissue change, the chronic stage.

The **chronic stage** appears in the iris as dark gray or dark yellow. This represents an even lower metabolic rate in the organ, again with an even greater decrease in blood, lymph and nerve activity. The immune system at this stage is now so weakened that it cannot resist or fight against disease. Body functions are very slow to react, toxins are not eliminated adequately and fatigue occurs. The body organ is now very slow to react to treatment. For an organ to reach the chronic stage, it may take many years of poor diet and living habits. If the chronic condition is not brought back into the active acute stage, the organ will degenerate.

The **degenerative stage** is seen in the iris as a disappearance of superficial fibers so that only the microscope is able to view the lowest level and the area appears nearly black. This represents the stage when the body no longer has the strength to heal itself. This is a condition that is difficult to reverse or treat such as arthritis, cancer, diabetes etc.

The **final stage** occurs when an area in the iris is totally black. This stage is rarely seen as it represents death of the tissue and irreversible damage. This is a stage where there is no longer tissue activity, but inactivity. It is now impossible to save the organ or group of cells. The cells have been deprived of nutrients for too long.

The body is a miraculous self-healing organism, and in the chronic stage it can reverse disease but once it reaches the degenerative stage, the disease becomes stronger than the regenerative capability of the organ. This is not to say that there is no hope when a patient has reached this stage in one or more of his organs, but the chances of recovery are greatly diminished. Often, at this point I recommend very drastic measures and changes in lifestyle and eating habits so that the irreversible stage is not reached. What is wonderful about the human iris is that with modern technology today, I am able to determine at what general stage of tissue change an organ is and monitor changes that occur with time. In this way, I can assess whether treatment is working for my patients and whether their organs are becoming healthier.

What we must come to realize is that we cannot afford to let our bodies reach a stage of degeneration, where the possibility of irreversible damage can occur. We must not mask our symptoms with the multitude of suppressing drugs that are available in society only to see chronic disease crop up later in life. We must cleanse, nourish, and strengthen our body so it will be able to reverse itself and go back to an acute stage of activity, where the elimination of infections and accumulated mucus can place us back on the road to health. In my opinion, the only way to accomplish this task is to live a drug-free life with healthy nutritional habits and a minimal amount of stress.

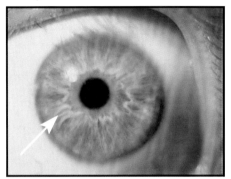

Acute stage

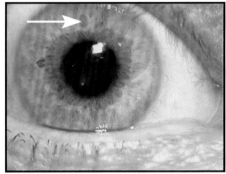

Pre-chronic stage

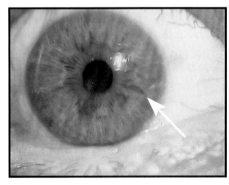

Chronic stage

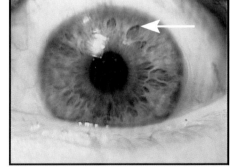

Degenerative stage

The Healing Crisis

I want to explain a very remarkable sequence of events that the body seems to go through on the journey to its return to health. As I hope you have come to realize, very few individuals are really truly healthy and very few who are being treated for medical problems will really become cured. The return to health is not as easy as popping a few pills until the symptoms go away. The return to health requires all living tissues to go back through the stages of tissue change until complete regeneration has been achieved. This means that an organ that is in the degenerative stage must first go back to the chronic, then the pre-chronic and finally, the acute stage in order to return to health. In iris diagnosis this gradual transition of body tissues can actually be seen in what we have described in the 5 stages of tissue change. But what do we mean by the healing crisis? Perhaps, some of you may recall the time when you started a new diet or a new cleansing program that you experienced some unpleasant physical effects. Many people often complain about changes in their complexion like acne, boils or skin rashes when they changed their diet for the better. On a vitamin or supplement program occasionally negative reactions occur such as those mentioned as well as aches and pains, runny nose, fever, nausea, and fatigue. What is really happening? Why is this person experiencing negative health effects when he or she is making positive health changes? This is what is called the **healing crisis**. Usually it only lasts for a few days at a time but it often occurs many times on the road back to true health. I am convinced that it is a necessary evil that everyone must go through if he or she really wants to be totally cured and free from disease.

I believe that when people go through a healing crisis, they are actually passing back through one of the stages of tissue change where the body is often trying to rid itself of harmful waste products and acidity in the form of phlegm, and discharge. This is occasionally too much of a load on the cleansing organs so feelings of fatigue and sickness occur as well as possible skin problems, indicating the need to rid the body of accumulated waste products.

The problem with most people is that as soon as some of these negative reactions occur, they run to the doctor for a prescription that prevents the level of tissue activity from getting to the acute stage. The patient is relieved of his symptoms right away but the condition will only come back again and the core of the problem will not be resolved. Everything that the body does, it does for a reason. We can't fool our bodies with temporary measures like superficial treatment with drugs; we can as I have mentioned before, only fool ourselves. The healing crisis should be looked upon as a positive not a negative event. With each healing crisis, the body comes closer to achieving true health and healing.

When you start a new health program that includes exercise, foods rich in nutrient value, a healthy low stress lifestyle, or food supplements to complement the diet, look forward to a number of healing crises along the way. With each step the body can eliminate in a natural drug-free way the toxins and waste material that have accumulated over the years. This, I believe, is the only truly natural way to achieve a complete cure of one's health problems. Believe in the body. It has amazing regenerative powers that even the greatest medical minds of today still can't understand and maybe never will.

Believe that with each healthy lifestyle change you make, the body will respond in a natural way and start to regenerate its tissues and organs while at the same time eliminating toxins and wastes along the way through one of many healing crises. Look forward to your next healing crisis because as your organs and tissues reach the acute stage of tissue change, you are getting closer to achieving true, optimum, and lasting health.

Chapter 9

The Pupil

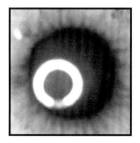

"The pupil — from total darkness we can uncover some light."

- **Pupil size, pupil displacement, pupil and ruff zone size, pupil flattening, ellipsoid pupils, pupil borders**

As we begin our analysis of the eye, we are drawn to the very center we call the pupil. What is the pupil? To many it appears as just a black spot in the center of the eye. The average person may vaguely understand that the pupil contracts under bright light and dilates in dim light, but to the experienced iridologist, the pupil unveils a whole world of important information about the patient. In the medical profession we know that the pupil is under control of the autonomic nervous system, both the sympathetic and parasympathetic. Our sympathetic nervous system takes control under periods of stress and our body reacts with an increased heart rate, breathing, and adrenalin flow as well as contraction of the radial muscles, which dilate our pupils. Our parasympathetic nervous system does the opposite and controls circular muscles which contract and constrict the pupil. Advertisers are very much aware of pupil size and often test the responsiveness of how pupils dilate to various visual stimuli to see what will attract the buyer. We know that pupil size also responds to a variety of emotions including excitement, excessive fatigue, and fear as well as to sounds, smells, and tastes.

The pupil is a hole through which light passes to the retina of the eye where our visual information is processed and sent through nerves to our brain. This hole will vary in size depending on the amount of light or whether we require near or far vision. Pupil size can also be affected by excess alcohol where pupils may dilate, certain drugs that can cause extreme contraction or dilation and even biochemical imbalance such as a lack of Vitamin B that lowers nerve tone. Patients who have suffered a stroke may have pupils that do not respond to bright light in the normal way.

Listed below are deviations that can be seen from the normal pupil and what they reveal, including pupil size, pupil displacement, pupil size in relation to ruff zone size, pupil flattening, ellipsoid pupils, and irregular pupil borders.

Pupil Size

Some extreme conditions of variation in pupil size are described below.

1. Miosis

Miosis is a term used to denote extremely contracted pupils indicating that the parasympathetic nervous system is dominant. When this condition is seen there may be bradycardia or slow pulse, excessive sex drive and a greater requirement for quality nutrition.

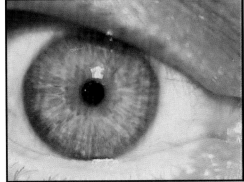

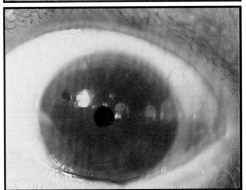

2. Mydriasis

When the pupils are abnormally large this signifies a condition called mydriasis where the sympathetic nervous system is more dominant. Associated with this condition are often tachycardia or fast pulse, low sex drive, poor appetite, and a high metabolic rate requiring greater amounts of vitamins and minerals. These patients may also suffer from bowel and stomach problems, urinary tract infections, and respiratory difficulties, which are often related to stress.

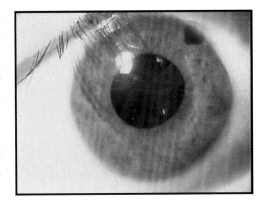

3. Anisocoria

This condition occurs when one pupil is remarkably different in size from the other. It usually results from blows to the head, extreme psychological stress, or may indicate disease or weakness on one side of the body.

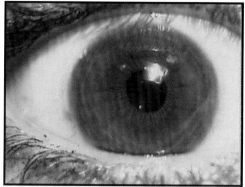

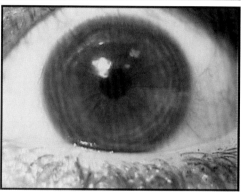

4. Hippus

Hippus denotes a condition where the pupil can change rapidly between miosis and mydriasis. This indicates that a considerable amount of stress is being placed on the nervous system and there is an imbalance between the sympathetic and parasympathetic nervous systems.

There are certain implications in regards to psychological behavior that these four conditions above represent which will be discussed in the chapter, The Brain, Psychological behavior and Iridology.

It is important when making a diagnosis from the pupil that one understands first what a normal pupil should look like.

The normal pupil is not exactly in the middle of the iris but slightly off center towards the nose and slightly higher towards the upper part of the eye. Normal pupils are perfectly round and of the same size, generally around 4 or 5 mm. in diameter. Any major deviations from this normal state indicate an abnormal state.

Pupil Displacement

We have already discussed how pupils can vary in size. The next indicator in pupil analysis is the location of the pupil in the iris. Pupils can sometimes be found closer to the side (medial or lateral), or to the top or bottom of the iris (superior or inferior). These pupil displacements have been associated with digestive, respiratory and heart, kidney, liver or spleen problems depending on where the pupil is displaced.

Pupil and Ruff zone size

There is a relationship between the size of the pupil and the size of the ruff zone. While the pupil size is indicative of the autonomic nervous system, the ruff zone size indicates the digestive capacity and degree of nutrient utilization. People with large pupils are more under control of the sympathetic nervous system and use greater amounts of energy less efficiently. Those with small pupils are under greater parasympathetic control; use less energy, more efficiently. There are four combinations that are possible when we consider pupil size and ruff zone size:

1. Large pupil size and large ruff zone size

These people have a larger capacity for food but often have a sluggish digestive tract and low enzyme production. They suffer from fatigue and reduced endurance as wastes from a slow metabolism accumulate.

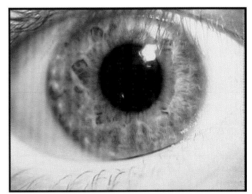

2. Large pupil size and small ruff zone size

The small ruff zone means that there is a lower capacity for digestion and small meals eaten more frequently are better for this kind of person. There is also reduced endurance as energy is rapidly used up.

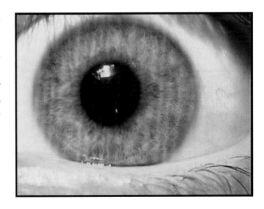

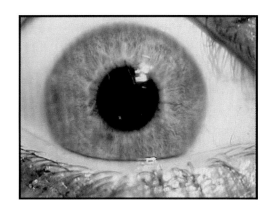

3. Small pupil size and large ruff zone size

These people have a great capacity and requirement for food but have poor energy utilization. They have great drive but poor endurance.

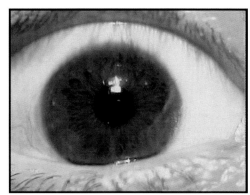

4. Small pupil size and small ruff zone size

This type is also suited to small meals due to the small ruff zone but energy stores are very high as well as endurance. They have a lot of drive and ambition, which can often stress the adrenal glands and affect the circulation.

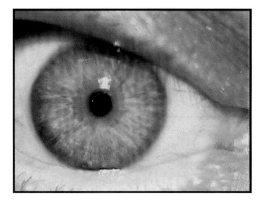

Pupil flattening

Pupil flattening reveals both physical problems and psychological tendencies. The psychological inferences are left to another chapter. Analyzing the pupil for specific flattening is a very useful method for diagnosing spinal problems and their effects on related organs in the body. Take a look at the Iridology Chart to the black pupil area and the white octagon inside.

1. A **superior flattening** can indicate a problem of the C1 vertebra as well as psychological problems discussed in a later chapter.

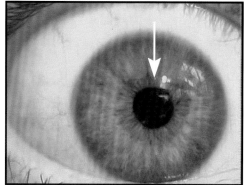

2. An **inferior flattening** indicates problems in the sacrum or coccyx, lower limbs, pelvic organs and often conditions like flat feet. Other problems may include knee and hip problems or headaches.

3. A **medial flattening** indicates problems in the thoracic spine. Related problems can include asthma, bronchitis, respiratory problems, and a weakened enervation to the lungs affecting breathing.

4. A **lateral flattening** reveals similar problems to the medial flattening with the additional weakness in the intercostal muscles between the ribs and diaphragm.

5. A **superior lateral flattening** indicates problems in the cervical spine often with shoulder and neck pain. Special consideration to hearing problems and balance is also indicated. Absentmindedness and cases of sleepwalking are sometimes seen.

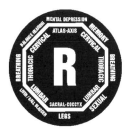

**Pupil flattening
Right Eye**

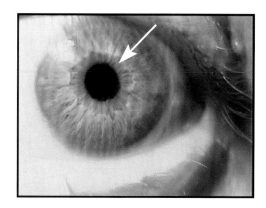

6. A **superior medial flattening** reflects problems in the cervical spine especially C1 and C3 vertebrae. Weaknesses in visual perception and memory can often occur.

7. **Inferior medial flattening** refers to disturbances in the lumbar and lower spine, sexual problems like impotence, and weaknesses in the bladder muscles.

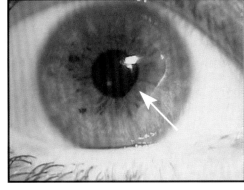

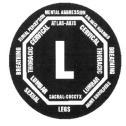

Pupil flattening
Left Eye

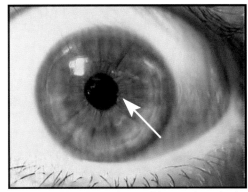

8. **Inferior lateral flattening** indicates thoracic and lumbar spine problems where in the right iris it can affect the liver and gall bladder functions. When seen in the left iris as well, this means there can be movement problems or pain and fatigue in the arms and shoulders.

Ellipsoid Pupil shapes

1. Vertical ellipse

Pupils that are vertically ellipsoid often show disturbances in acid-base balance, poor circulation and an increased cerebrospinal fluid pressure, which may affect mood and character.

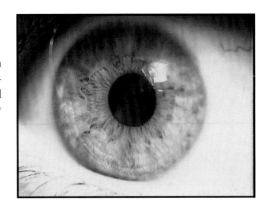

2. Horizontal Ellipse

This sign has been associated with severe fatigue, thyroid problems, respiratory distress, depression, and headaches.

3. Ellipse pointing to the left

This sign indicates a predisposition to stroke, crippling of the left side of the body, or impotence.

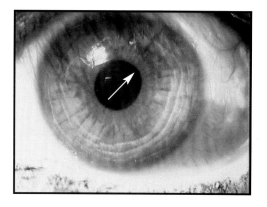

4. Ellipse pointing to the right

Problems can include paralysis of the right side of the body, bladder complaints, hormonal problems with menses or early menopause, and circulation problems.

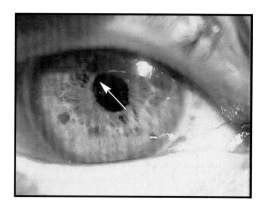

5. Ellipse pointing to right and to left

This sign indicates fluctuations in blood pressure, hearing problems, and memory problems with an increased risk of stroke.

6. Ellipse pointing to left and to right

This type can exhibit pain and spasms in the lower legs with bladder and bowel problems.

7. One sided ellipse

Asthma or breathing difficulties due to nervous causes can be associated with this sign.

Irregular pupil borders

The final sign that can be analyzed on the pupil is the border itself. A healthy pupil border is usually perfectly round with no breaks or thickenings or extra colors. Any changes to this normal border may indicate health problems.

A **thick leathery, brown pupil border** often indicates problems in the stomach, poor nutritional practices, and difficulties with the absorption of nutrients.

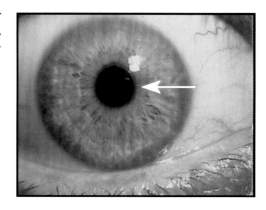

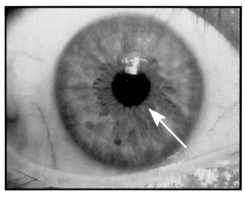

A **rough, notched pupil border** often indicates a weak spine and skeletal structure and joint problems or arthritic conditions.

Patches of gray on the pupil border can sometimes signify atherosclerosis and senility.

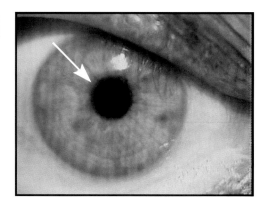

Well, I hope it can be appreciated now that the pupil is not just a black dot in the middle of the eye but an encyclopedia of information owing to the fact that its function is connected, as is our iris, to our complex integrated nervous system. Again, it is always important to remember not to take any of the pupil signs alone and make a diagnosis but use what they reveal along with other signs in the iris and sclera to come up with the most accurate analysis.

All the organs and systems in our body are related to each other for, as you will see, the signs in the iris, pupil, or sclera constantly overlap and can confirm your initial hypothesis.

Chapter 10

The 6 Essential Processes of Life

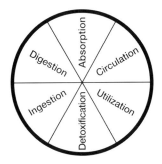

"Your body is your shrine, your sanctuary, it is the vehicle that carries your soul on the long journey we call life. If you give it what it needs, it will reward you with the realization of all your dreams."

Before we get into the different systems in the body and how iridology can assist us in reading their signs in the iris, I want to mention some of the essential processes that our body must carry out in order to maintain health or to combat disease. We often make the mistake and look only at the patient's specific problem area. This error will not occur in iridology if we always learn to look for the cause of the disease and not just signs that indicate symptoms. Look at the body holistically as it is composed of a number of systems all working together to accomplish a smooth and efficient operation of all our daily activities. I have identified six essential processes without which healing of disease or regeneration of body tissues cannot occur. If any one or more of these processes is weakened or malfunctioning, the entire organism suffers.

If we believe that our body depends on quality nutrients for its existence then the initial process of **ingestion** is critical. We can look at ingestion holistically as nutrients are not only the foods we eat but also the air we breathe, the energy we receive from the sun or other sources around us, the love or happiness that life brings us, or the spiritual fulfillment that nourishes our soul. These are all essential nutrients for us to maintain physical, psychological, and spiritual health.

Take a look at the foods we eat. Many are full of chemical preservatives, additives and colors. Our diets are extremely high in sugar and fat. Are these really nutrients that we want our bodies to process? Remember we are what we eat. Whenever we process foods in any way including freezing, canning, or microwave cooking, valuable nutrients are lost. Most foods today do not have the quality of nutrients that we imagine.

The oxygen that we need to feed each one of our cells is often inadequate. Pollution, smog, smoking, carbon monoxide from cars, stress, these all reduce the quality and quantity of vital oxygen that we need. Without oxygen we die. Our cells become prone to disease.

The energy from the sun for production of Vitamin D, and various forms of energy around us such as friendship, love, and nature, are all vital nutrients.

Our spiritual lives are often incomplete and the need to find out why we are here and really what our task is in life are questions that each one of us must come to terms with at some time in life. Are we really happy? Is it possible to be physically healthy when we are under stress or suffering from depression? I don't think so. Sooner or later our physical bodies will begin to suffer.

So the process of ingesting all the right nutrients every day is for each one of us the basic crucial starting point in the maintenance of our health.

As we will learn in the chapter on the intestines, **digestion** is a process that breaks down the nutrients from the foods we ingest into basic components including fats, sugars, and amino acids. Our body requires fats, carbohydrates, proteins, vitamins and minerals but just because we ingest them in our diets, does not mean that they will be absorbed into our bloodstream. The process of **absorption** of nutrients depends on a lot of factors. The environment in our digestive system must have the right pH or acid base balance and this depends on the quality of bile produced in the liver and stored in the gall bladder, the digestive enzymes secreted by the pancreas, and the intestinal micro flora. In current times the number of people with weak livers, insufficient enzyme production, and unbalanced micro flora, is growing rapidly. As a result, less of these vital nutrients get across the intestinal membrane into the transportation network of our circulatory system.

Circulation is one of the processes of the body that we often take for granted. Without a strong efficient heart that can pump the nutrients through our vast network of veins and arteries, our cells would starve. Our blood vessel walls need to be strong and flexible to maintain stable blood pressure and stay clear of fats and cholesterol deposits that are often evident in many heart condition problems. We often forget the importance of exercise and diet to support and maintain our circulatory system.

So far, we have traced the essential nutrients that we initially ingest right through to where they have entered our circulatory network. Their ultimate destination is our cells, but the process of nutrient **utilization** will determine whether the cells take up these nutrients or not. There are many factors including our hormonal system controlling the efficient utilization of our nutrients.

Through the process of metabolism, waste products and toxic substances are constantly being produced and these must be removed from the body through a number of **detoxification** channels. These include our colon, kidneys, the liver, lungs, lymphatic system, and skin. If any of these elimination organs are weakened, the toxic load in the body is increased. The increased toxicity in the body will lead to a variety of conditions including fatigue, headaches, and skin problems, as the cells of the body begin to function at less than optimal capacity. The health of the body is now in a very weakened state and serious diseases have the potential to develop.

I call these the six essential processes of life. Remember them well as you begin your journey into the investigation of the iris. If you always keep them in mind as you search for clues to the cause of a patient's problem, you will have the greatest chance of success in your diagnosis. They have assisted me over the years as a reminder to constantly view the body as a whole set of integrated systems.

Chapter 11

The Digestive System and the Leaky Gut syndrome

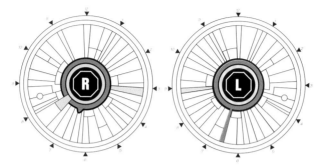

"Without the proper functioning of the digestive system, nutrients cannot get to the cells to maintain health."

How important is our digestive system to our health? Can the eye unlock some of the mysteries to the condition of our digestive system?

It is my opinion that the digestive system is undoubtedly the most critical system in our body. The digestive tract consists of the mouth, tongue, salivary glands, esophagus, stomach, small and large intestines, rectum, and anus. Organs associated with digestion are the liver, gall bladder, and pancreas. The digestive system is one of the cleansing systems in the body, ridding it of unwanted wastes. In this way it acts as part of the immune system. The main functions of the digestive system are digestion and absorption of food and water, destruction of the harmful bacteria that we ingest, production of vitamins by the intestinal flora and elimination of waste material. Of all the systems in the body, I believe the digestive system suffers most from our modern unhealthy lifestyle, poor diet, drugs and the antibiotics we ingest. Diseases associated with the digestive system include; allergies, malabsorption syndromes, colitis, Crohn's disease, constipation, diarrhea, heartburn, excess gas and meteorism, diverticulitis, Leaky Gut syndrome and many others.

Take a look at these diseases. Many cannot be cured with modern medicine and the others? Ask yourself how many drugs you have taken to relieve stomach problems, constipation, allergies etc.

We need to start to take care of our digestive system. It is like the motor in our cars, we need to feed it with the proper fuel. Some experts on ageing say that each of our digestive systems has a genetically determined number of times that it can digest meals. This means that if we eat 3 times a day for approximately 80 years this amounts to about 88,000 meals. Some mice if fed less food live far longer than mice fed all they can eat. This could mean that if we as humans ate less, we would be able to add more meals and therefore more years to our lives because our digestive system would last longer.

While we often think of our digestive system's only function being the breakdown of food to its basic elements, we often forget that it is not only a question of what foods we eat to achieve adequate nutrition, but also how we digest that food, and whether it is absorbed into the blood.

The process of digestion begins in the mouth where enzymes begin to break down some carbohydrates. In the stomach, pepsin and hydrochloric acid are necessary to break down proteins into smaller units.

The acidic environment of the stomach is also crucial in destroying dangerous bacteria that we ingest with food so that they don't go further and get into our blood system. People with a lack of hydrochloric acid in the stomach cannot digest proteins very well and are susceptible to bacterial infections. In this way our digestive system is our first immunity defense. If it is not in good working order we may begin to have diseases that are related to our stomach and intestines although we may not be aware of this.

Stress also affects stomach acids and digestion. Movement of food through the digestive system is crucial. People who have a rapid movement through a short digestive tract often cannot absorb enough vitamins and minerals into the blood so they need to eat more often. This is seen in the iris as a small ruff zone ring around the pupil. Peristalsis depends on a number of factors. Why do we have constipation? There are three main reasons. We don't drink enough water, we don't have enough fiber in our diets, and we don't exercise. Other factors include a deficient nervous system, poor circulation, and unbalanced intestinal micro flora.

The liver and gall bladder also play an important role in the production, storage and concentration of bile, which is needed for the efficient digestion of fats.

Often when the liver is weakened, the quality and quantity of bile produced is insufficient, leading to digestive problems. The formation of gallstones due to changes in bile pH can impede bile flow and drastically affect our digestion.

Our pancreas has the function of secreting digestive enzymes. A healthy pancreas prevents us from having the feeling of excess gas and bloated stomach after eating.

The micro floral environment within our intestines is an area that is under great study. Within our intestines exist hundreds of types of bacteria, some beneficial and some detrimental to our health.

The rampant and irresponsibly widespread use of antibiotics is compromising the healthy micro floral environment of our intestines and is creating a host of contemporary diseases that classical medicine cannot cure. Furthermore, bacteria are becoming resistant to the antibiotics that we are using so we find that many of these drugs are not effective any more. What is modern society's answer to this problem? Manufacture even stronger antibiotics, which will further damage our digestive system. We need to start thinking differently. Instead of trying to kill the viruses and bacteria that give us disease with drugs, we need to be strengthening our immune system in order that our body can battle to prevent disease in a natural way.

When healthy micro flora are absent, the unhealthy bacteria can damage the intestinal walls and toxins can leak into the blood and generate free radicals that may cause problems from over-active or under active thyroids to allergies, asthma, migraines and arthritis. Further, we are less able to protect ourselves from disease, since a healthy intestinal wall is the first line of defense in our immune system. It is no wonder that I usually see a poor digestive system when I look at the eyes of cancer patients.

If our digestive system is not working properly, our whole body is affected. If we cannot absorb vitamins and minerals, proteins, fats and carbohydrates into the blood, we cannot expect to cure a disease elsewhere in the body. That is how crucial a healthy digestive system is to our state of health.

The area of the digestive system in the eye is often referred to as the "ruff zone" which is the first major zone encircling the pupil. The innermost ring of this zone is the stomach and the outer ring, the small and large intestines, are found encircling the stomach zone. This zone in a healthy patient is generally approximately one third of the distance from the pupil to the iris border, indicating a healthy balance between the autonomic nervous system and the digestive and absorptive capabilities. When the bowel becomes constricted, digestion and absorption become limited. A person with this kind of problem is better suited to eating smaller meals more often to achieve the daily requirements that the body needs. As the bowel balloons, there is loss of muscular tone, reduced peristalsis and increased transit time in the bowel. Bowel enlargement may often be seen with those who suffer from constipation. We may also see conditions like an over acidic stomach, lack of stomach hydrochloric acid, diverticula in the intestines, growth of harmful bacteria, poor absorption of nutrients, weakened intestinal walls, ulcers, reduced peristalsis, diminished nerve supply, pressure of organs on the digestive system as well as many other stomach and intestinal disorders.

The Leaky Gut Syndrome

I pay special attention to this area because as I mentioned before, every patient I have had who has a serious terminal disease always has a malfunctioning digestive tract, leading me to believe that the source of the problem lies there. Earlier I mentioned how the micro floral environment in our intestinal tract is crucial as our first line of defense. If this environment becomes disrupted a free radical cascade occurs due to what is now referred to as the Leaky Gut syndrome. What do we mean by a free radical cascade? Well, many of you have probably heard about free radicals and how we really don't want them because they slow down our cells and weaken our bodies. If we expose the beneficial micro flora in our intestines to antibiotics, drugs, chemical preservatives and other toxic substances, they are destroyed, and the non- beneficial bacteria start to proliferate. This creates a host of problems including damage to the intestinal walls and the leaking through of harmful toxins into the circulatory system. Our immune system is then triggered to react and begins to fight these unknown substances entering our bodies and free radicals are produced. If our intestinal flora is not replaced our intestines become a breeding ground for free radicals and our digestive and absorptive capabilities are drastically diminished. The result is, a free radical cascade that can damage cells and organs, promote arthritis in joints, affect glands like the thyroid, and lead to a reduced level of immunity in the body. I see this problem today in at least 80 percent of my patients and it has now reached almost epidemic proportions. Even children often display the Leaky Gut syndrome and it is no wonder as they inherit digestive weaknesses from their parents combined with the rampant use of antibiotics. This often leads to allergies or skin problems like eczema.

Our intestines suffer greatly from the host of preservatives, colorants, and food additives that are present in our foods today along with the number of drugs and antibiotics we consume. We must realize that without a healthy intestinal wall, we cannot absorb nutrients effectively, and no health problem can be cured if our organs do not receive adequate nutrition. Natural healing begins with the intestines and what we feed ourselves day after day.

You may have often heard the saying, "You are what you eat" but that is not completely true. You are what you absorb and you need a healthy digestive system to be in the best of health.

Intestines - iris examples

1. Healthy balanced ruff zone

2. Constricted ruff zone- indicating limited digestion and absorption

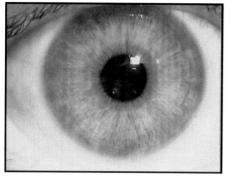
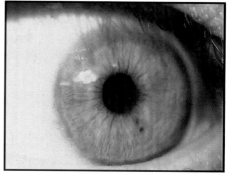

3. Ballooned bowel- loss of tone in colon, reduced peristalsis, constipation

4. Obscured ruff zone- toxic bowel

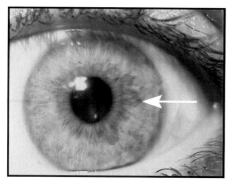
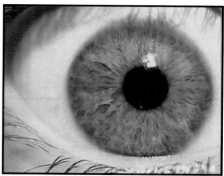

5. Diverticula- trapped fecal material

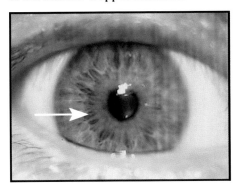

6. Jagged ruff zone- nervous system causing diarrhea or constipation

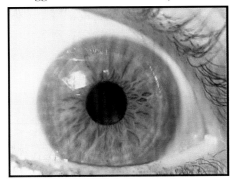 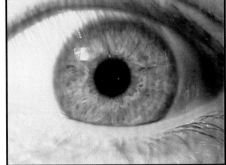

7. Prolapsed transverse colon

8. Absorption ring- lowered absorptive ability in intestines

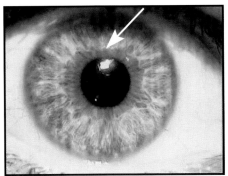 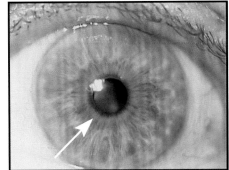

9. Over-acid stomach

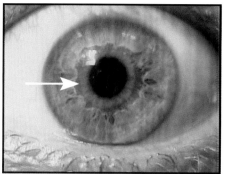

10. Under-acid stomach

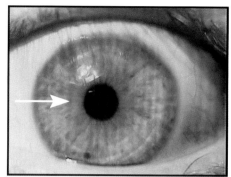

11. Ulcers

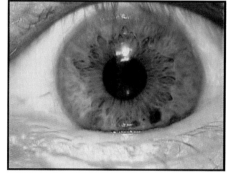

12. Leaky Gut syndrome

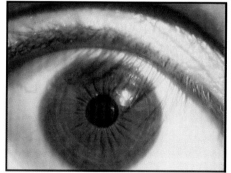

13. Insufficient pancreatic enzyme production

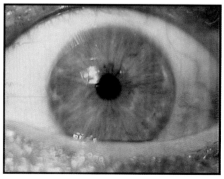

14. Poor quantity or quality of bile production

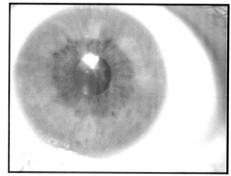

Chapter 12

Detoxification organs and Iridology

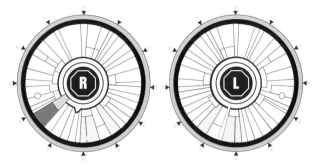

"Detoxification is the key to a clean, healthy body and a clear mind."

In a previous chapter we have already discussed one elimination organ, the intestines. In this chapter we will learn about five other detoxification organs that assist in the elimination or detoxification of toxins and waste products in our body. Many diseases occur as a result of increased toxicity in the blood and tissues due to inefficient or faulty detoxification organs.

I cannot stress enough, how important it is for us to rid the body of toxins and my belief is that their accumulation in the body slows down cell function and increases the chances of cancer formation or serious chronic degenerative conditions.

The Kidneys and the Urinary System

How important are the kidneys to our health? They are extremely important and it is a shame that we so often neglect them. Perhaps we don't know enough about them in order to make the necessary changes or don't realize that we can make those changes ourselves without the use of drugs to improve their condition.

If I told you that if everyone's kidneys were healthy, there would be no more wars, no more negative thinking, no more anger, jealousy, depression, anxiety, theft, or violence, you obviously wouldn't believe me, but could there possibly be even a little truth to it? Think about it. What do our kidneys do? They cleanse our blood. I strongly believe that our physical health greatly affects the way we interact with people around us, as well as the way we feel psychologically. We may not be able to end all wars or hatred in the world, but I am convinced that abuse of our kidneys contributes to negative energies that we build around ourselves. Let's take a look at these two important organs that lie inside our bodies.

The kidneys are bean-shaped, paired organs, which lie in the posterior abdominal wall, one on each side of the vertebral column. They are responsible for filtration of the blood and removal of waste products by producing urine. Each kidney is composed of approximately one million filtering units, called nephrons. The kidney is supplied with about 1.2 liters of blood of which about 125 ml. is filtered into the nephron each minute resulting in a total filtrate volume of about 180 liters a day, of which only 1 or 2 liters is removed from the body as urine.

This shows how intricate and precise filtration through the kidney needs to be. The kidneys regulate the water content of our body's internal environment, as well as its acid-base balance. The kidneys remove wastes from the body including the drugs we take and chemical preservatives in food that we ingest. The kidneys are vital to our health. Without them our bodies would become so toxic that we would die. We take them for granted. Unlike the liver, however, they do not regenerate easily and once diseased they create a number of health problems.

How can we tell that we have weak kidneys? Often patients with kidneys that are not functioning optimally are those with dark rings or bags under their eyes or who suffer chronic fatigue. In the iris of the eye, those who are born with a kidney lymphatic constitution type are prone to kidney problems and if not careful end up on dialysis in later years. Many iris signs also indicate weak kidneys associated with urinary tract problems and bladder infections. Through my years of iris studies, I have found that kidney problems or disposition to kidney problems can be detected as early as three years of age. It is very important to assist weak kidneys as soon as possible to prevent serious degeneration that is then difficult to cure. Another possible outcome of weak kidney function is skin problems. This includes eczema, dry and itchy skin, boils and various other skin diseases. Poor kidney function also often manifests itself in fluid accumulation in the body, or edema. This can be seen as puffiness in the face, fluid accumulation in the arms or legs, or in the head where migraine headaches often occur. Yes, even migraine headaches can often be traced back to a poorly functioning kidney.

We need to be reminded to take care of our kidneys. Feeling tired, angry, anxious, depressed, nervous, or aggressive, may be a sign that our bodies are overloaded with toxins.

Another important lifestyle observation that I have made is the water that is consumed by most people on a daily basis. Our bodies need water for every chemical reaction that occurs within them. We cannot live without water, yet I constantly hear from patients that they don't drink enough. Every one of you out there needs a minimum of 1.5 liters of water a day. Our kidneys need water to properly get rid of the toxic wastes in our bodies and to reduce the risk of kidney stone formation. Water does not include alcohol, coffee or black tea. If you suffer from arthritis, back pain, fatigue, or headaches, you cannot expect to improve your health if you do not drink enough water! So many health problems that I have seen have improved dramatically once the body is supplied with one of the most important and essential nutrients we need constantly every day, plain unsweetened and un-carbonated water.

While iris diagnosis often detects a weakened kidney, it also can reveal the consequences such as skin problems, toxin accumulation in the body, over-acidic conditions, high blood pressure, and the strain on other organs such as the liver and the heart. Kidney stones cannot be seen in the iris of the eye as they have no nerve supply but often acute inflammation signs may be seen in the kidney areas, which can indicate the possibility. As we saw in the kidney lymphatic genetic iris constitution, yellow pigment in the iris can indicate weaknesses in the kidneys and the appearance of breaks in the fibers, flecks, lacunae, or nerve rings can be seen in conditions like glomerulonephritis, bladder infections, and other associated urinary or kidney problems.

The location of the kidneys on the iris map is in both irises, the left kidney in the left iris just before 6 o'clock to almost 6:30 and in the right iris from about 5:30 to just after 6 o'clock. The urinary bladder is found in the right iris between 4:30 and 5 o'clock in the right iris and between 7 o'clock and 7:30 in the left iris. These areas are marked in yellow on the iris map.

The following photographs indicate weaknesses in the kidneys, or the urinary bladder.

1. Kidney weakness in right eye– chronic

2. Kidney weakness in left eye

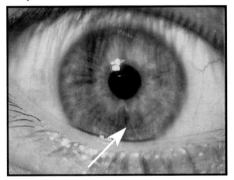
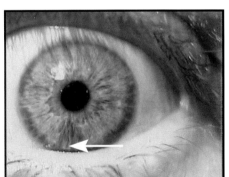

3. Urinary bladder- acute condition

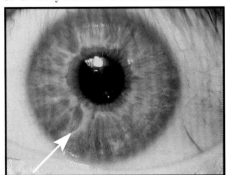
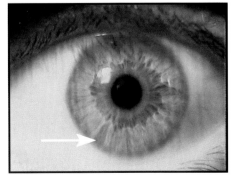

4. Kidney lymphatic genetic constitution   **5. Lacunae in kidney area**

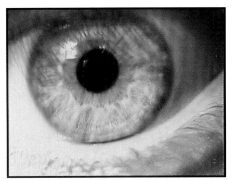
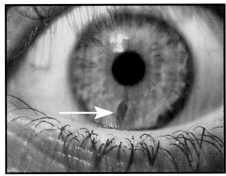

6. Kidney tumor   **7. Kidney stones**

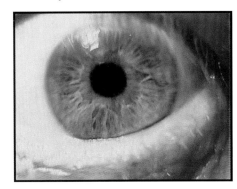
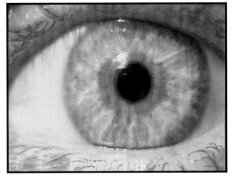

The Liver

The liver may not be the most glamorous organ in the body but it is the largest and in my opinion, the second greatest in importance next to the intestines.

While we speak with respect when we talk about the heart or with great concern when we mention the almighty kidneys, the liver almost seems to be a subject of distaste, only slightly less embarrassing than the bowels.

Everyone is aware, however, that alcohol in enough quantity will damage the liver. The liver is often a topic of discussion at parties where alcohol is being consumed. It is unfortunate though, that this is generally the extent of most people's understanding of this organ.

When the liver is not functioning properly, people feel cranky, nauseous, and irritable and symptoms range from flatulence, headaches, fluid retention, skin problems and constipation to jaundice and cirrhosis. People need to realize that if they take care of their livers, they will solve a great majority of their health problems, since it is the liver where the problems often begin. The liver performs around 22 primary functions and is responsible for a total of two thousand reactions and functions in the body. Think about it for a moment, almost 2,000 functions from one body organ, such is the importance of our liver.

While the liver is a integral component of the digestive system in its production of bile, it has many other functions including metabolism of hormones, fats, and carbohydrates, synthesis of plasma proteins, formation of urea which is eventually filtered by the kidneys and removed as urine, destruction of worn-out blood cells, and glucose balance. One of its primary functions is detoxification of the blood.

With our current lifestyles, present environmental pollution, prevalent nutrient deficiencies, and over-processed and chemically contaminated foods, it is no wonder that our livers suffer. It is impossible for the liver not to have an effect on our overall health. With the consumption of thousands of chemical additives present today in foods plus the ingestion of so many prescription drugs, the need for detoxification is far greater than it has ever been.

It is a rare individual today who has a perfectly functioning liver and this consequently means that women are producing children who start their lives with liver problems. It is not surprising that many parents are concerned when their children are picky eaters who refuse to eat protein foods. When the liver is not healthy, people find it difficult to handle animal protein. The protein deficiency then creates further health problems and consequently other systems in the body begin to malfunction. The result is a population that is very lethargic, with no appetite in the morning, which needs to be artificially stimulated into activity with coffee and sugar or cigarettes in order to make it through the day.

A variety of vitamin supplements and herbals can assist our liver to regenerate so that it can handle the excessive loads of toxins that are imposed upon it and thus prevent problems in the future.

As mentioned before, the iris often reveals liver involvement by brown flecks seen throughout the iris. The liver itself can show weakness signs. On the iris map it is located in the right iris between 7:30 and 8:00 right next to the gall bladder.

1. Cirrhosis of the liver

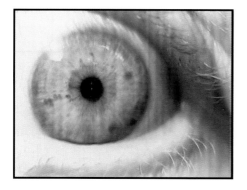

2. Drug spots

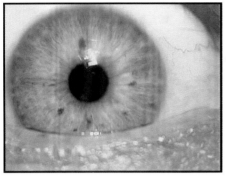

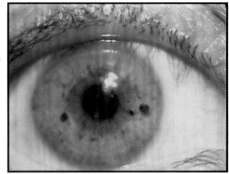

3. Liver weakness

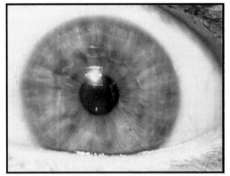

4. Toxic load on the lymphatic system due to liver weakness

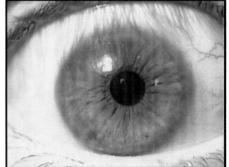

5. Inflammation of the liver

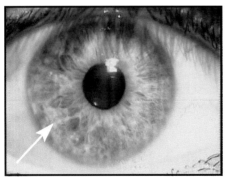

6. Sclera sign of liver problems—fatty liver

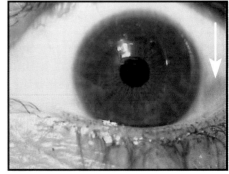

7. Liver tumor

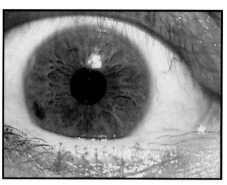

8. Nerve rings –liver area

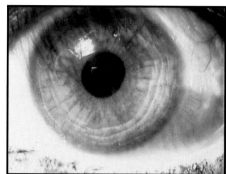

9. Liver congestion—liver transversal

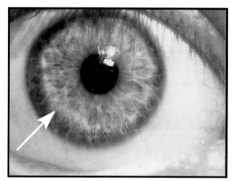

10. Gall bladder

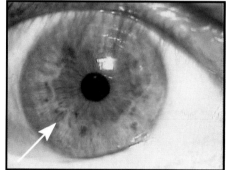

Lungs

The respiratory system, one of the most important detoxification channels in the body will not be discussed here as it is given special attention in the following chapter.

The Lymphatic System

Do you suffer from constant coughs, sore throat, or flu? Do you find that the frequency of these conditions is increasing every year? Are bacterial infections taking longer to clear up? If the answer is "yes", you probably have a congested lymphatic system.

The majority of my patients accept these conditions as normal and the incidence of cold symptoms or flu a few times a year is taken as nothing to really be concerned about. However, the body is showing signs of weakness and responds by raising body temperature to destroy bacteria, and discharging from the nose to rid the body of its increased toxic load, as we find in the common cold.

The lymphatic system is like our second circulatory system. It is a specialized system of one- way valves which carry lymph, a clear fluid that is produced in the tissues and which empties into major blood vessels. The main purpose of the lymph fluid is to direct toxic substances like bacteria that have escaped the blood vessels to lymph nodes where they are filtered out and inactivated by lymphocytes. It can be referred to as our garbage disposal system in the body.

Another function of the lymphatic system is to absorb fats from the intestine.

If the person suffers from the Leaky Gut syndrome and large molecules of fat cross the intestinal border, the lymphatic system can become blocked or congested, reducing its ability to detoxify the body.

You may have recognized your lymphatic system during an infection where the body becomes overloaded with toxins and major lymph nodes such as those found under the armpits, the groin or neck begin to swell.

The lymphatic system is therefore an important part of our immune system.

Other organs associated with the lymphatic system are the appendix, spleen and tonsils. When the tonsils are removed, the ability to remove toxins is diminished and the rest of the lymphatic system becomes over-burdened.

In the iris, the lymphatic system is found as a ring around the outer iris next to the skin zone. On the iris map it is shown in red. It is in this area that I frequently see a ring of clouds known as the lymphatic rosary. These clouds are often white, indicating an acute condition and if chronic they show up as yellow, orange-yellow or brown clouds. They may not encircle the entire iris but may show up in sections indicating congestion of the lymphatic system in that area of the body. Frequently associated with lymphatic clouds are weaknesses in the intestinal walls or in any of the other detoxification organs.

Treating the digestive system and other elimination organs will reduce the toxic load and congestion in the lymphatic system and improve immunity.

I often use the Bowen method of massage to initiate adequate drainage into the lymphatic ducts due to an overly congested lymphatic system.

Examples of congested lymphatic systems in the iris are included below.

1. Lymphatic rosary–acute   **2. Lymphatic rosary—chronic**

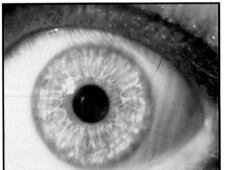
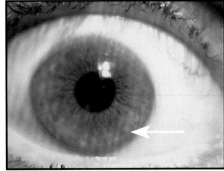

3. Lymphatic rosary only in specific section of iris

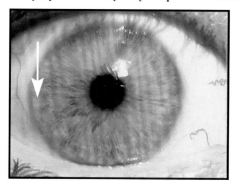

The Skin

The final detoxification organ is our skin. This is an organ on which most of us spend unbelievable amounts of money. We buy expensive creams, lotions, acne solutions, anti-aging formulas, moisturizers, suntan lotions, and deodorants. It is unfortunate that many of these formulas are chemical substances that block the sweat glands and prevent the elimination of toxins.

Very often chronic skin diseases such as eczema or acne are suppressed when treated with ointments that contain antibiotics or corticoids. A healthy skin requires that all the detoxification organs operate at one hundred percent capacity. This means that the kidneys, liver, lungs, lymphatic system and digestive system all contribute to clean, healthy skin. When toxins accumulate in the body to the point where these organs cannot cope, they find their way out of the body through the skin. The result can be chronic skin infections that recur from time to time or even last for years. Creams and ointments are only superficial treatments. The real cause is the body's inability to eliminate toxins and that is what must be treated. A variety of vitamin supplements and herbals can assist in regeneration and improvement of function of the detoxification organs. In my practice, I have seen many skin conditions disappear once these principles are followed.

The skin also requires good circulation so that the smallest blood vessels, the capillaries, can transport wastes to the sweat glands for their elimination.

Sunlight is necessary for the production of Vitamin D, while exercise and a healthy diet and lifestyle will ensure that the organs of elimination work to their full potential.

Drinking enough pure clean water, skin brushing, and allowing the skin to breathe by wearing natural materials, will assist in the removal of accumulated toxins.

In the iris the skin zone is found as the outermost ring labeled in pink.

Often the rim around this part of the iris is darkened indicating accumulation of toxic material because of inadequate elimination from the skin. Toxic clouds or haze are also often present in this area, revealing skin problems like eczema, dermatitis, dry itchy skin or other chronic skin conditions. Like the lymphatic rosary, the skin signs may sometimes be seen in only some parts of the skin zone ring, indicating skin problems in that area of the body.

1. Eczema

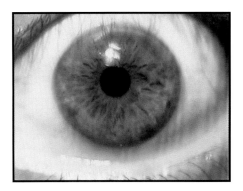

2. Dark skin rim

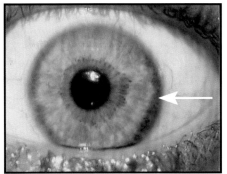
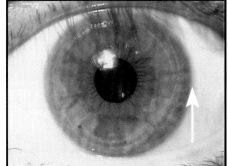

3. Toxic haze and clouds in the skin zone

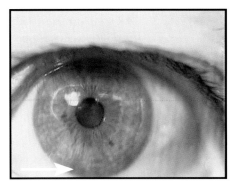

Chapter 13

The Breath and River of Life

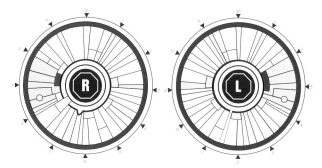

"The respiratory and circulatory system - The breath and the river of life."

The Breath of Life

When was the last time that you really took a look at how you breathe? In practice I see many patients with very weak diaphragms and breathing muscle signs in their irises. I believe the reason is that most of us don't really know how to breathe properly. We take it for granted. If you take a look at most people in the city who are under stress, their breathing is very shallow. It is no wonder that they suffer from chronic fatigue and headaches. The amount of oxygen they inhale is low, not to mention that pollutants in the air like carbon monoxide from cars or cigarette smoke reduce their percentage of oxygen intake.

We need to go back to the basics. Think of how natural it is to take a deep breath when we are in a park or a forest or in the mountains where there is an abundance of nature. I need to apply this to the urban, city environment. I like to recommend at least 5 minutes of deep-breathing exercises every day, to strengthen the breathing muscles and increase the intake of oxygen.

Smoking is one of the most damaging practices to our respiratory system. The tar and toxins that are found in cigarettes are poisons to our bodies. As we know the accumulation of these toxic effects are seen in the frequency of lung cancers found among smokers.

Degenerative iris signs in the lungs or inflammation of the bronchi and bronchioles are always seen in heavy smokers. Often the effect is also seen as weakened heart function and circulation problems like varicose veins or hemorrhoids.

Our lungs need an ample supply of clean fresh air to maximize oxygen exchange and uptake into our cells so that all our metabolic processes can function effectively. Our lungs in the process of respiration exhale carbon dioxide, one of the prime waste products of cellular metabolism. As we know from the previous chapter, the lungs are one of the detoxification organs so they are critical in the elimination of waste.

Why are there so many breathing problems like asthma and bronchitis?

There are many factors that may contribute to this problem such as smog, pollution, and allergies to chemical additives in foods, milk products, poor breathing practices, low immunity, and greater susceptibility to infections.

Our society is plagued by colds, runny noses, and coughs, for which we immediately run to the local drugstore to find a tablet or cough syrup. We are not anxious to find out why we suffer from these conditions, only how we could temporarily stop the symptoms.

My personal opinion is that we will never find a cure for the common cold because it is not a disease. I believe that the common cold is a reaction of the body to eliminate toxic waste products. When our noses are running, when we get a fever, when we start to cough, or when our head starts to pound, these are all indicators revealing that we are run down. Our immunity is weakened, we are more susceptible to disease and our body needs to get rid of excess toxins. It is a mistake to stop this process through the use of cold preparations or other drugs used to alleviate these symptoms. This only further suppresses the problem and blocks the elimination channels, which the body so desperately needs.

It is interesting to note that the respiratory system takes up a large portion of the iris map indicating its great importance to our health and well-being.

The respiratory system consists of the trachea, bronchi, bronchioles, lungs, pleura, vocal cords, and diaphragm. They are located in blue on the corresponding zones in the iris map. The breathing center representing the medulla is found in the brain zone in both irises. Strokes, brain tumors, or other diseases can affect the breathing center in the brain and can also lead to breathing difficulties and respiratory conditions.

Take care of your lungs. They allow the life-giving exchange of oxygen for the waste product carbon dioxide. They can be classified as an ingestion organ as well as an elimination or detoxification organ. All our metabolic processes depend on oxygen as well as all our thought processes. In this way our respiratory system is required for a healthy body and a peaceful, clear- thinking mind. It is our breath of life.

Some respiratory signs seen in the iris

1. Upper lung weakness

2. Inflammation of the bronchial passages

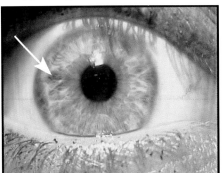 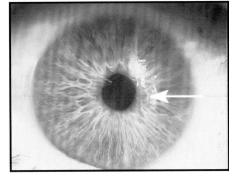

3. Weak diaphragm

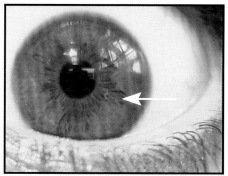

4. Inflammation of the pleura

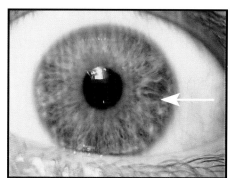

5. Inflammation of the vocal cords

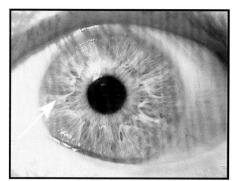

6. Chronic bronchitis

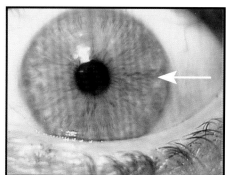

7. Effects of smoking

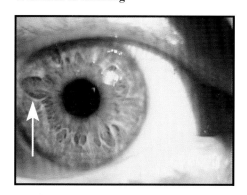

The River of Life

Being one of our six essential processes of life, our circulatory system is critical to our health and survival. It is central to our existence in mind, body and spirit. In the physical sense, we need our heart to pump blood throughout our bodies to nourish our cells and to remove wastes. The heart in other words gives us an abundant source of energy. In the emotional and spiritual sense, the heart represents our feelings, our intuition and unselfish behavior. As we begin a new millennium, I hope that we can learn to give from the heart and be kind to one another. Each one of us has something to share, or something to contribute for we are all special in our very own individual way.

What do we mean when we talk about the circulatory system? The heart, which lies between the sternum and the spine slightly to the left of the midline of the body, is central to the circulatory system. It is a magnificent pump whose endless effort propels blood through a vast network of veins, arteries and capillaries. The heart feeds every single cell of our body with oxygen and nutrients. These same nutrients, vitamins, and minerals are required by the heart itself to keep it healthy and strong. The heart of a mouse beats about 1000 times per minute, an elephant's 35 - 40 beats per minute, and a whale's 15 times per minute. An adult human heart beats approximately 60 - 80 times per minute. Healthy blood pressure is around 120/80. High blood pressure is generally evident when the systolic pressure, the higher number, is greater than 135, although the diastolic pressure, the lower number is often considered more important if it is higher than normal for a specific age group.

Our circulatory system is one of the most neglected systems in our body. It is no wonder that the top causes of death in Western societies are circulation and heart related. Think of the number of people with heart attacks, angina pectoris, arrhythmias, high blood pressure, low blood pressure, anemia, atherosclerosis, arteriosclerosis, varicose veins, and hemorrhoids. Do you believe that these conditions are all inherited? Perhaps we are raising children who start life inheriting our circulatory weaknesses but they can to a large extent be overcome. The majority of these problems can be reduced or eliminated with diet and lifestyle changes.

How can we expect to have a healthy heart and circulation if we don't exercise? When we exercise regularly, our resting pulse decreases, showing that our heart is becoming stronger and more efficient in pumping blood through the body. The body was never made to be transported by cars and elevators and to sit for endless hours watching television. It was made to be active and productive. We can see how quickly the body deteriorates when patients lie in a hospital bed for only a few days. So important is exercise, that I stress it to all my patients whether they are 8 years old or 80. We cannot use age as an excuse. Take for example the mighty Hunza people. Many of them who live up to 120 years are often found still walking over fifty kilometers a week! I have also met many older fit people who are 70 years old and have blood pressure of 120/80!

We cannot neglect the incredible effect that stress has on our heart and circulation. It can influence our heartbeat, weaken the heart muscle, create fluctuations in blood pressure or cause cardiac arrhythmias. I see this most often occurring in the blue neurolymphatic constitution and the brown hematogenic iris type when there are stress rings. However, it can occur in any constitution.

Overeating, excess tea, coffee, alcohol and smoking all affect the heart in a negative way. Emotions such as grief, negative thinking, and anger place a great strain on the heart as well.

In the iris of the eye the heart is seen on the left side around 3.00 o'clock. In this zone marked in red, it is possible to see iris signs that may reveal cardiac arrhythmias, and damage to the left side of the heart muscle, which can predispose the patient to dangers of heart attack or angina pectoris. The heart zone is also located in the right iris between 9 and 10 o'clock. This is because the heart lies in the center of the body, slightly to the left. The right part of the heart is indicated in the right iris. Conditions that affect the right side of the heart can include venous problems like poor venous return or congestion in the veins or lungs.

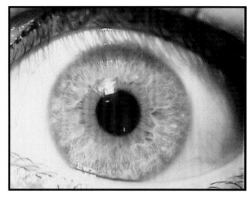

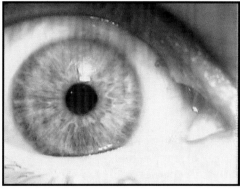

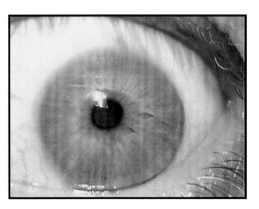

It must be remembered that other signs in the iris, not only in the heart area can indicate potential circulation problems.

A very common sign that we have already seen, especially in elderly patients is the "arcus senilus," a white ring around the outside border of the iris. This sign indicates arteriosclerosis (hardening of the arteries) and often appears several years before a heart problem is recognized. This is another reason why regular iris diagnosis is recommended to alert the patient of potential health problems. When the arcus senilus ring extends to other areas around the iris like the heart and respiratory zone, a cholesterol ring is formed and this can be found to affect the coronary arteries. Examples of these conditions were displayed in the chapter on fundamental iris signs.

When the veins and arteries are carrying blood full of toxins, due to a clogged lymphatic system, we often feel fatigued and become sick. Our immune system is revealed in several ways in the iris, one of which is a lymphatic rosary around the periphery of the iris. When these clouds are dark, they indicate that our lymphatic system is allowing toxin-laden lymph to enter the circulatory system. The blood and lymphatic circulation as they work together are located in red in one of the outer rings of the iris.

The sclera or white of the eye as we will see, reveals a number of signs in the form of blood vessels that indicate a variety of health and circulation problems. These include varicose veins, hemorrhoids, poor elasticity of the veins and arteries, arteriosclerosis, high blood pressure, anemia, decreased circulation to the periphery and many other circulation disorders. A detailed summary of these signs is in the chapter on signs in the sclera.

Lack of oxygen in the blood indicating lack of exercise or iron anemia is often seen as a blue ring encircling the iris on the iris/sclera border.

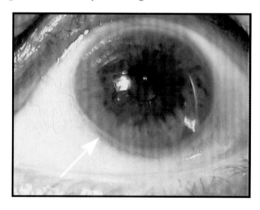

As always, do not forget the effect that other organs have on the heart and circulatory system. Look for signs in the digestive system, the lungs, the kidneys, and the liver, all of which are often associated with related heart or circulation problems.

A certain respect or admiration must be given to the role of the circulatory system, as it connects every organ and cell in the body. It transports messages in the form of hormones, oxygen from the lungs, and nutrients from the digestive system, in the form of blood to every living cell of the body. All of the processes, that keep us living, breathing, working, thinking, and creating, depend on this wonderful intricate system, our circulatory system, the river of life.

Chapter 14

The Hormonal System and Reproduction

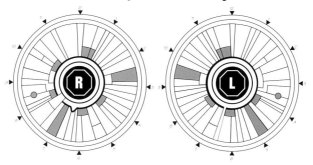

"*Hormones are necessary for regulation of body functions and reproduction.*"

What is the hormonal system? What are hormones?

While the blood and circulation are our internal transportation system, the hormonal glands are the regulators of the body. What are hormones? Hormones are substances that the endocrine glands secrete which are then transported by the blood and end up at specific target tissues. These hormones work together with the nervous system, the main communication system in the body and they regulate and affect many of the body's functions.

Remember, hormones are needed for growth and weight control, the menstrual cycle, water balance, blood sugar control, sexual characteristics, reproduction, the immune system, metabolism and many other vital processes. An unbalanced hormonal system will often lead to many health problems.

Why does our hormonal system become unbalanced?

Each of our endocrine glands responds to messages or information that is transported via the blood, circulatory system and the nervous system.

They secrete hormones depending on these signals. If our bodies are toxic and full of chemicals, drugs, and other artificial substances, our immune system can become overwhelmed and soon there is confusion in how these signals are interpreted. With the addition of the oral contraceptive pill, steroid use, and hormone replacement therapy, not to mention the countless drugs we ingest, it is no wonder that there are so many people with hormonal problems. There may be other causes including genetic defects or dispositions such as we have seen in the hormonal iris constitution, or tumors that cause pressure on the glands. Also, do not forget the effect that sugar has on our hormonal system. Large amounts of blood sugar can also interfere with hormones circulating in the blood.

In this chapter we will go over some of the glands that have hormonal action on the body, and whose signs can be seen in the iris. They include the pituitary, adrenal, pineal, thyroid, the pancreas, ovary, and the testes. They are colored orange on the iris map. All of these glands are critical to the coordination of numerous activities and work together to create a smooth functioning of all the body systems. An iris diagnosis is not complete if the hormonal system is not analyzed.

The Pituitary Gland - The Master Gland

Often called the master gland of the body owing to its vast control over many other endocrine glands and organs, this tiny gland weighing only about a half a gram lies under the hypothalamus. In the iris it is located in the brain zone just after 12 o'clock in the right iris and just before 12 o'clock in the left iris. The pituitary is actually composed of two glands, the anterior pituitary and the posterior pituitary. An outline of the major hormones that this gland secretes is described below. As you can see this miniscule gland is ex-

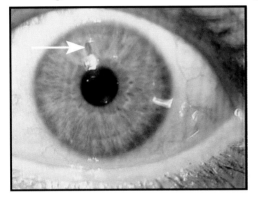

tremely important and any white signs in the pituitary zone can indicate inflammation of the pituitary, while dark signs including radii solarii, indicate weakness.

Any red signs along the radii solarii or throughout any part of the iris indicate pituitary involvement. Owing to its control over a wide range of body regions, pituitary signs can be seen in other areas of the iris besides just the pituitary zone.

Menstrual problems and Hormone Replacement therapy

One of the most common problems I encounter with female patients are problems with their menstrual cycles, including premenstrual cramping, excessive bleeding, or irregular cycles. Many use oral contraceptive pills to mask or suppress these symptoms but the real problem lies with their hormonal system, primarily the imbalance between the hormones that are secreted by the pituitary gland and the adrenal gland. Masking these problems can lead to infertility problems, endometriosis, and problems later in menopause. In my opinion, hormone replacement therapy used to prevent hot flushes and osteoporosis is not the answer either and its use is leading to an increase in cancer of the breast and uterus. The body must regain its own hormonal balance in a natural way. Look at the condition of the digestive system and the liver as well, as they contribute to the health of the hormonal system. Often there will be iris signs in these areas when the hormonal system is causing problems. A balance of good nutrition with vitamin and mineral therapy for better functioning of the pituitary and adrenal glands will usually correct the problem within a period of several months.

Anterior Pituitary

Hormones	Actions on the body
1. Growth hormone	– regulates the growth of tissue and bone
2. Thyroid stimulating hormone	– triggers growth of thyroid/hormones
3. Adrenocorticotrophic hormone	– stimulates adrenal gland/hormones
4. Follicle stimulating hormone	– promotes growth of ovum/spermatozoa
5. Luteinising hormone	– stimulates growth of sex organs/hormones
6. Prolactin	– causes breast development/milk production

Posterior Pituitary

Hormones	Actions on the body
1. Oxytocin	– stimulates uterus to contract during birth
	– causes mother's breast to release milk
2. Antidiuretic hormone	– controls water loss and urine formation

The Adrenal Gland and Stress

The adrenal gland lies on top of the kidney and is best known for its role in adrenalin release during times of stress. Since our modern living consists of considerable stress, this gland is frequently activated and thus, often becomes exhausted. Consequences of weakened adrenal glands due to constant and intense stress are lowered immunity, blood sugar fluctuations, loss of energy, and blood pressure changes. In the iris, the adrenal gland is located above the kidney zone at approximately 6 o'clock. Signs often include breaks in the fibers or lacunae at various stages of tissue degeneration. Often when there are weaknesses in the adrenal glands, look also for nerve rings in the iris.

Adrenal Gland

Hormones	Actions on the body
1. Steroid hormones (Adrenal cortex)	– control blood sodium content
	– regulate water metabolism
	– influence energy metabolism/blood sugar
	– affect sexual characteristics
	– speed up utilization of fats
2. Adrenalin and Norepinephrin (Adrenal medulla)	– raise blood pressure, heart rate and cardiac output
	– increase blood flow to muscles, liver, and brain
	– inhibit digestive system activity
	– increase conversion to glucose

95

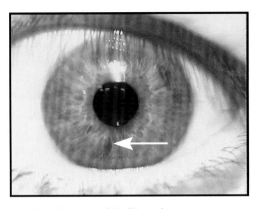

The Pineal Gland—Problems with Sleeping

The pineal gland, a minute pea- sized gland found at the base of the brain between the two hemispheres is located on the iris map right next to the pituitary gland in the sleep zone of the brain. It is one of the least understood of the endocrine organs but it has been demonstrated that it gathers information from every part of the body and it can control activities of the pituitary as well as other endocrine glands. One of the hormones it

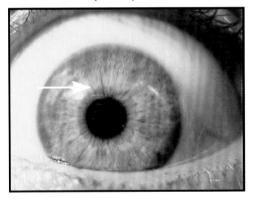

secretes is melatonin, an antioxidant that helps regulate our sleep-wake cycles, assists our immune system, and plays a role in calcium metabolism. A compromised pineal gland has been linked to bone diseases like osteoporosis.

As in the case of the pituitary gland, there are often radii solarii in the iris, deep channels that run through the pineal gland as well as clouds, separation of fibers and lacunae. These all indicate a weakened functioning of the pineal gland.

The Thyroid Gland— Metabolism Regulator

The thyroid gland is located at the front of the neck and secretes the hormones thyroxine, and calcitonin. In the iris, the thyroid gland is located between 2 and 3 o'clock in the right eye and between 9 and 10 o'clock in the left eye.

The thyroid gland is vital for regulating the metabolism of the body. An under functioning of the thyroid (Hypothyroidism) often leads to a slowed metabolism, hair loss, coarse dry skin, sensitivity to cold, weight gain, bradycardia (slow pulse), moodiness, inability to handle stress, lack of sexual interest and lower energy levels. There is also a greater chance of atherosclerosis as reduced thyroid secretion leads to increased levels of cholesterol in the blood. A patient with this condition also shows slow healing ability.

An under-active thyroid is identified as a gray lesion or lacunae or separation of fibers in the thyroid zone.

An over-functioning thyroid (Hyperthyroidism) often leads to increased metabolism, weight loss, tachycardia (fast pulse), hyperactivity, goiter (enlarged thyroid gland), nervousness, increased appetite, and protruding eyeballs. In the iris this condition is often seen as a white lesion or white fibers in the thyroid area and/or a bird's beak lacuna, which can be seen in any part of the iris.

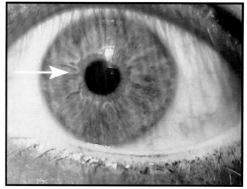

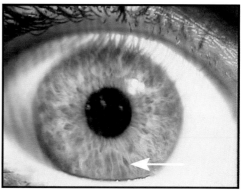

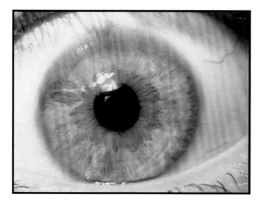

Thyroid problems are also often indicated in the iris as beige or misty orange-yellow pigment throughout the iris.

The parathyroid glands located just behind the thyroid regulate calcium and phosphorus metabolism in the body. Lesions or lacunae in the thyroid zone can also indicate weaknesses in the parathyroid glands but these signs should be used only as an approximation as they are often not reliable.

Thyroid Gland	
Hormone	**Action on the Body**
1. Thyroxine	– increases rate of energy and heat production – speeds up protein, carbohydrate and fat metabolism – promotes growth and maturation
2. Calcitonin	– lowers blood calcium by depositing it in bones

The Pancreas— Blood Sugar Regulator

The pancreas is located posterior to the stomach and connects to the duodenum. It has a dual function. It secretes pancreatic enzymes into the duodenum for digestion as well as secreting the hormones, insulin and glucagon. These hormones are responsible for the regulation of blood glucose levels.

A lower level of blood glucose (hypoglycemia) will stimulate the release of the hormone glucagon, which will act on the liver to release glucose, thus raising the blood sugar.

A higher level of blood glucose (hyperglycemia) will stimulate the release of the hormone insulin, which acts on the liver and muscle to store glucose, thus lowering the blood sugar.

In a healthy person, these hormones will never allow the blood sugar to rise or fall to dangerous levels. If there are disturbances in the function of the pancreas, or in the utilization of insulin, then conditions like hypo or hyperglycemia, as well as diabetes can occur.

Diabetes

It should be mentioned at this point that the incidence of diabetes is growing alarmingly fast. I believe this has a lot to do with our diet and lifestyle. More and more patients are showing iris signs indicating blood sugar fluctuations, weaknesses in the liver and pancreas, adrenal gland exhaustion due to heavy stress, and dysfunction of other endocrine glands such as the pituitary, and thyroid gland. These factors all contribute to the increased incidence of diabetes today. Our daily intake of sugar and sugar products is extremely high, creating a load with which the pancreas cannot keep up and the abuse of our livers is often forgotten in its role as a regulator of blood glucose. As we have seen, the adrenal gland, thyroid gland, and pituitary gland also influence the activity of the pancreas.

Signs of diabetes include glucose in the urine, high blood glucose levels, excess urine production, excessive thirst, and weight loss. Associated with diabetes are kidney and circulation problems, as well as cataracts.

Blood sugar fluctuations also affect our energy levels and our mental or psychological health state. Often seen are depression, anxiety, irrational behavior, and hyperactivity, which in children commonly result in poor attention span and difficulties at school.

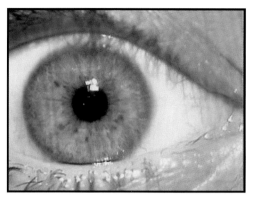

The pancreas areas in the iris are at 4 and 8 o'clock in both irises and are seen occasionally at 10 o'clock in the right iris. As we learned in the chapter on colors, the color orange in the iris often signifies pancreatic involvement.

This color may appear anywhere in the iris and can sometimes be orange-brown. If seen in the ruff zone, it usually involves the pancreatic enzymes, while outside the ruff zone, fluctuations in blood sugar. Look for lacunae in the pancreas zones as well as violet coloring in the ruff zone, which can often mean dispositions to blood sugar problems, including diabetes. Sprinklings of orange color around the outside of the ruff zone also indicate problems in glucose metabolism.

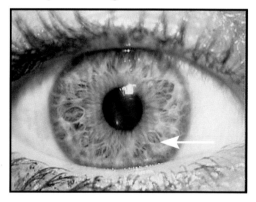

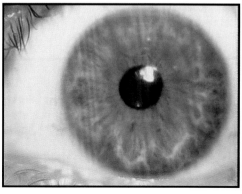

The Ovaries -- Estrogen and Progesterone

The ovary is also an endocrine gland as it secretes the sex steroid hormones, estrogen and progesterone. The ovaries working in conjunction with the pituitary gland maintain the female cycles of ovulation and menstruation. Estrogens are needed to prime the breast for milk secretion, to initiate and maintain secondary sex characteristics, and to prepare the uterus for embryo implantation by acting to increase its inner lining.

The main task of progesterone is preparing and maintaining the lining of the uterus for embryo implantation until the placenta hormones take over.

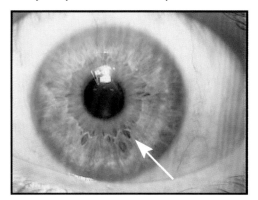

Imbalance in hormones secreted by the ovaries or problems with the ovaries themselves can be seen as lesions in the ovary zones, located at 7 o'clock in the right iris and 5 o'clock in the left. Look also at the adrenal gland and the pituitary gland zones. Sometimes a red lacunae or red pigment indicating pituitary involvement can also be seen with problems associated with ovarian hormone production.

The Testes— Testosterone

The testes, which are also under the influence of the pituitary, produce the male sex hormone, testosterone. Testosterone is required in production of sperm, secondary sex characteristics, and muscular development and growth.

The testes are located in the same zones of the iris together with the ovaries. Problems with the testes and hormone production are usually seen as lacunae or separation of fibers.

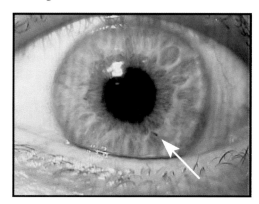

The Reproductive Organs

The reproductive organs include the uterus, breast, vagina, penis, and prostate gland. The ovaries and testes have already been discussed.

It is important to mention that pregnancy cannot be seen in the iris, as it is a natural process.

The vagina, penis, uterus, and prostate gland are shown in yellow and found in a sector of the iris map just before 5 o'clock in the right iris and just before 7 o'clock in the left iris. The vagina and penis occupy the lower half of the sector while the prostate and the uterus occupy the upper half of the sector near the ruff zone.

The breast is located in orange in the respiratory zone between 8 and 9 o'clock in the right iris and between 3 and 4 o'clock in the left iris.

Lesions or signs in the vagina, penis, uterus or prostate gland are often white inflammation signs, which can indicate infections or discharges, pain, burning sensations, impotence, or enlargement of the prostate gland.

Lacunae in these areas especially if dark in color often indicate more serious conditions which include infertility problems, prostate gland problems, or serious degeneration as in cancers or tumors.

Separation of iris fibers or lacunae formation in the breast areas can indicate predisposition to cyst formation or breast cancer. I have seen this occur most often in the Neurolymphatic constitution although it can be seen in any of the other types.

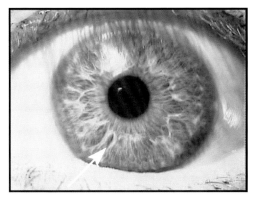

Uterus

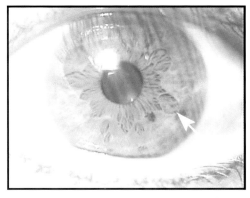

Cyst in the breast

Chapter 15

Bones and Muscles

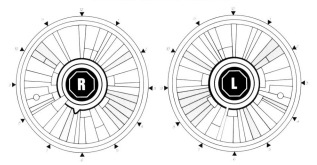

"The bones and muscles - the structural framework of the body."

Our structural system, which gives us our shape and size, consists of bones and body muscles. What we often forget when we think of the human skeleton is that it is composed of living tissue which is constantly being replaced and regenerated. Our skeleton represents an enormous store of calcium and phosphorus and hormones like the parathyroid hormone and calcitonin regulate the movement of these elements into and out of the bone. Our bones are also the sites of red blood cell formation; they protect our spinal cord, brain, and vital organs, and provide an attachment for muscles, tendons, and ligaments, which enable our bodies to move.

Just as the other organs in our body, the human skeleton also relies on adequate nutrition in order to perform the above functions. A poor diet combined with problems in the digestive system can easily result in deficiencies in calcium or minerals that are required for healthy bone structure. The outcome is a number of bone conditions including osteoporosis and arthritis. Obesity also contributes to a major stress on the spinal column and is often associated with back pain and joint problems.

Lack of exercise and poor posture also affect the density and strength of our bones as well as the condition of our muscles, contributing to a weakened skeletal system, joint and ligament problems and curvatures of the spine. Once our muscles cannot adequately hold our spinal column in the correct anatomical position, the spine is subject to frequent injury and a slight twist or irregular movement can often result in backaches or serious back pain. Spinal problems can also create migraine headaches, and affect our moods and behavior. Pinching of nerves due to weakened vertebrae can affect communication of nerve impulses to our organs and muscles in the entire body, affecting their function.

The skeletal system is shown in green on the iris map and consists of the sacral, lumbar, thoracic, and cervical spine and scapula indicated in both irises, from just after 3:00 to 4:30 in the right iris and 7:30 to almost 9 o'clock in the left iris. The cervical vertebrae and neck area can be seen at 10:30 in the right iris and 1:30 in the left iris. Just below this area are also located the clavicle and shoulder. The ribs are located in both irises below the lower respiratory region. The pelvis can be found before 7 o'clock in the right iris and before 5 o'clock in the left. The jaw is seen in the right iris at 2 o'clock and in the left iris at 10 o'clock. The skull is located in the brain zone and the bones of the arms and legs are located at 8 o'clock and 6 o'clock in the right iris, and 4 o'clock and 6 o'clock in the left iris, respectively.

Another area of the eye that can be used to assess the condition of the spinal column and the health of the joints, as we have learned previously, is the pupil border. Its numerous types of flattening and signs relating to the spine can be found in the chapter on the pupil.

The muscular system, although not directly indicated on the iris map, is associated with each part of the skeletal system and problems in the muscles are found in their respective skeletal area. For example, the intercostals, the muscles between the ribs, are found in the rib zone on the iris map.

Remember that the degree of weakness or degeneration of the spine and muscular system can be observed according to whether the iris sign in the area is acute, pre-chronic, chronic or degenerative. The degree of pupil flattening is also an indicator of the seriousness of the condition. Often acute back or muscle pain is revealed as white streaks or clouds in the spinal areas of the iris.

While the majority of patients turn to pain killers, chiropractors, physiotherapists, and massage therapists, often a prescription of regular exercise, good posture, enough water, and adequate nutrition is all that is needed to strengthen bones and muscles, lubricate joints, and improve circulation. This will dramatically improve the condition of the musculoskeletal system and prevent serious problems in the future.

1. Lumbar spine

2. Neck

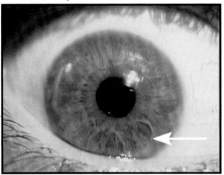 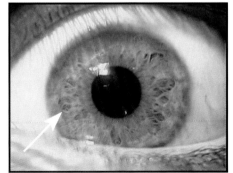

3. Arthritis

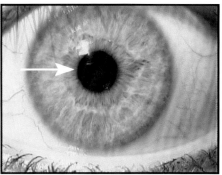

4. Legs

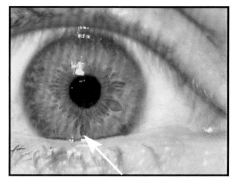

5. Shoulder

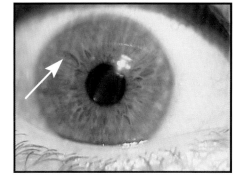

6. Jaw

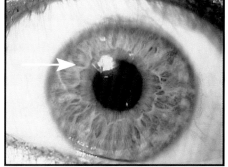

Chapter 16

We see, we smell, we hear, we touch, we taste

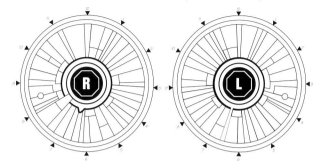

"The senses are our contact with the world around us."

Sensory organs

Our sensory organs, those that enable us to gather information about the world around us are magnificent gifts of nature that bring us the sense of pleasure, protect us from harmful occurrences, and gather information from which we send to our brains to process as images, smells, tastes, feelings, and sounds. It is hard to imagine a life without our sensory organs. Just envisage a life without sounds like music, without the tastes of your favorite foods, the smells of perfume and freshly baked bread or the touch of another human being.

Our sensory organs, our eyes, ears, noses, our tongues, and our sense of touch connect us to the outside world. Without them we would be quite alone in a shell, without interaction with the outside environment. The majority of us take our senses for granted but we immediately feel isolated when our phones are disconnected or we can't get through and connect to the Internet. Just imagine a life without sensory organs. Those who have lost their sight, speech or hearing abilities can appreciate how their lives can be affected. This does not mean that the loss is always negative since many who have lost their sight have gained heightened abilities of their other senses. These people may thus be equipped with skills a normal person does not have. The next time you see a blind person or one who can't hear, take the time to think about the value of your senses.

What about our sixth sense, or our sense of intuition? While this sense cannot be quantified or seen in the iris of the eye, it does exist. There are some who rely on this sense to guide them through life, or point out advantageous opportunities that may arise. Many employers use their intuition when hiring personnel rather than the classical method of sorting through resumes and interviewing prospective employees. People often get a good or bad feeling when they meet a person for the first time. Sometimes when they listen to reason rather than intuition, they are badly mistaken and an unfortunate experience may follow. I believe we all have this sixth sense, but perhaps we just don't know how to use it yet. We use our sense of intuition whenever we react to our feelings or subtle promptings.

The eyes—the windows to our souls

People, who have never heard of iris diagnosis, often associate investigation of the eyes with an eye check-up for possible glaucoma or quality of eyesight.

When what the examination consists of is explained, people often ask if their eye problems can be seen directly by looking at the eye or by looking at the position of the eye in the iris, according to the iris map. An eye doctor will assess the condition of the eyeball and structures, test the intraocular pressure, and assess the eyesight. What can often be visible are cataracts, which show up as cloudiness over the pupil, infections, pterygium (discussed in the chapter on the sclera), and direct injuries to the eye or structures around the eye.

The iridologist searches for reasons why there are eye problems. Often through the analysis of the iris, one will find that the cause of the eye problem is usually somewhere else rather than in the eye itself. Look for associated conditions with eye problems including nutritional imbalance due to digestive problems, blood sugar problems as in diabetes, high blood pressure or blockages in blood flow to the eye, high blood cholesterol, damage to the nerves or nervous system, or under-active hormonal glands. Certain drugs such as corticosteroids may also be the cause.

Just as every organ has its place in a certain segment of the iris, so do the organs of the eye. They are found in the frontal head region between 1 and 2 o'clock in the right iris and between 10 and 11 o'clock in the left iris. The nose is also found in this region next to the eye. The sensory organs have been labeled in light blue on the iris map.

In these areas only structural problems can be seen. Eye problems involving the nervous system and optic nerve may sometimes be revealed as signs in the sensory regions of the brain zone. Also, problems in visual perception can be seen when there is a superior medial pupil flattening, as we saw in the chapter on the pupil.

White signs in the eye zone can indicate inflammation as in conjunctivitis, or other infections or irritations, while lacunae and separation of iris fibers indicate weakness in the eye itself or degeneration of the lens, retina, cornea or other eye structures.

The nose, ears and tongue

The nose, as mentioned has its place next to the eyes in the iris map, while the ears are shown just before 11 o'clock in the right iris and just after 1 o'clock in the left iris. The tongue although not labeled on the iris map is usually found in the jaw zone next to the nose sector.

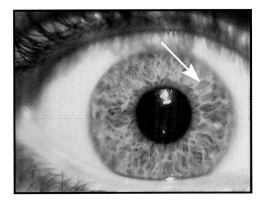

Nose

Weakness signs in these sensory organ segments include white inflammation marks in the nose, ear, and tongue areas indicating infections, inflammation or discharge. Degener-

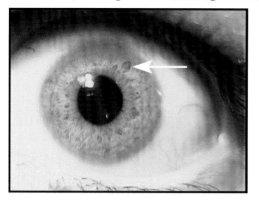

ative indications like lacunae or fiber separation in these areas once again indicate degeneration of the structures of the ear, nose, or tongue, which can include deafness, disorders of taste, and other nasal problems. Balance problems and hearing deficiencies can sometimes be seen in the balance center in the brain or as a superior-lateral pupil flattening.

Ear

Chapter 17

Signs in the Sclera

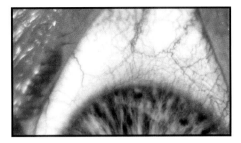

"The sclera is the vast white ocean surrounding the iris terrain. It too unlocks many secrets to the health status of the patient."

Although iridology strictly speaking is about the language of the iris itself, many iridologists forget that the sclera reveals a large number of signs that can guide or assist in achieving an accurate diagnosis. The sclera is the white of the eye and an iris diagnosis should always include a thorough examination of this area. As most signs in the sclera relate specifically to the circulatory system and considering that heart disease is one of the greatest killers in present day society, it is worth taking note of potential problems that may provide missing clues. Although signs in the sclera are sometimes random and vary in accuracy, they should be taken in context with the signs, colors, and general iris constitution to obtain a total picture of the overall health status of the patient.

Never make the mistake of taking only one sign and making a poor diagnosis. The experienced iridologist will take all signs into consideration before he or she makes the final diagnosis. Listed below are examples of various signs that are commonly seen in the sclera.

A. Vascular Signs seen in the Sclera

1. Allergy sign

This sign appears as small blood vessels that encircle the outside of the iris on the sclera and resemble a crown of thorns. The more evident is the sign, the more serious the allergic symptoms, which often include irritation of the mucous membranes and skin. This sign can be seen to overlap the iris itself indicating allergies to substances outside the body such as pollens and grass.

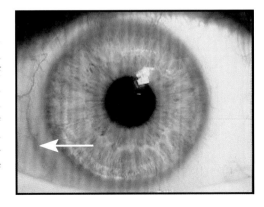

When seen only on the sclera, foods and ingested substances such as dairy or wheat products may be the cause of the allergy.

2. Meander and framed meander sign

These signs are found in any part of the sclera. The meander vessel as its name implies wanders in no specific direction. It represents connective tissue weakness primarily related to an insufficiency of the veins. Often an inherited sign, it can result in varicose veins, hemorrhoids, bleeding from the gums, or frequent bruising. Meander vessels that are faint usually indicate the possibility of spider veins. The framed meander includes a meander vessel surrounded by a straight vessel on each side. Like the meander vessel it also indicates a general weakness in the veins with possibilities of venous congestion and internal and external varicose veins.

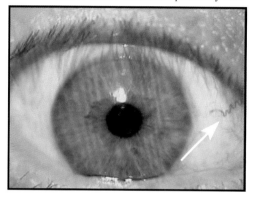

3. Migraine or Headache sign

This sign is similar to the allergy sign but confined to only the uppermost head area of the iris. When this sign is seen it is common for the patient to suffer from migraines or headaches.

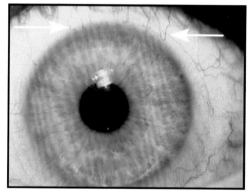

4. Porcelain vessel

These vessels found in the sclera are thick, bright, and raised vessels that stand out noticeably as they look as though they are made of porcelain. They indicate that there may be an impending coronary thrombosis or hardening of the blood vessels as in arteriosclerosis.

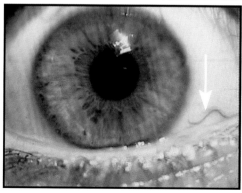

5. Spiral vessels

This sign is associated with decreased elasticity of blood vessels leading to abnormal changes in blood pressure. When these vessels show up faintly in the sclera they usually indicate low blood pressure while brighter signs indicate high blood pressure or blood pressure fluctuations.

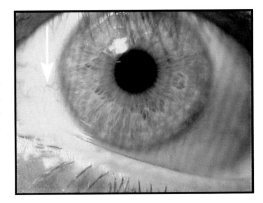

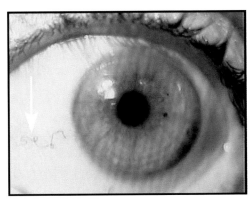

6. Pointing vessels

These are straight vessels in the sclera and they generally point to an adjacent area of the iris where there can be a potential health problem. They are usually found outside the

heart, liver, lungs or major organ areas where there may be chronic problems. The longer, the more visible, and the closer the pointing vessels are to the iris, the more serious the condition.

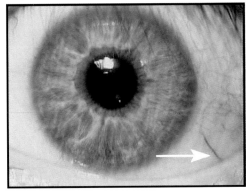

7. Tangent vessels

These vessels form a tangent to the outside of the iris and indicate congestion in the arteries or veins in the adjacent area of the iris. They are commonly seen in the heart, liver, spine, or brain areas.

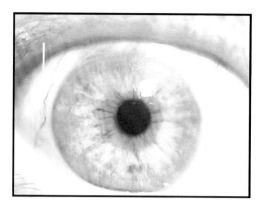

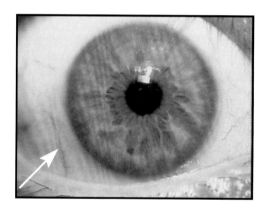

8. Trauma fork sign

This sign is seen as a single blood vessel that branches into two. Although not very reliable, it can sometimes suggest trauma or concussion that occurred at one time in life, to the area of the body that it runs adjacent to in the iris.

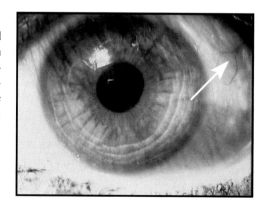

9. Vessel Branches

Vessel branches are small, thin vessels that stem off a large thick vessel.

They sometimes indicate anemia as well as high sensitivity to changes in the climate, especially cold and damp conditions, which can aggravate rheumatic symptoms.

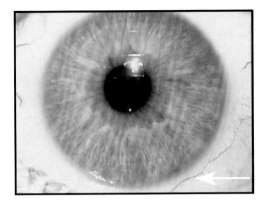

10. High Blood Pressure sign

A straight vessel with a bulge at one end may indicate a potential for high blood pressure or blood pressure fluctuations.

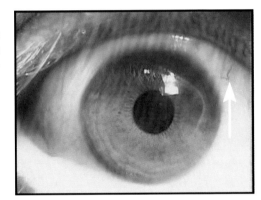

11. Protein sign

These are straight vessels that run down from the lower part of the iris into the sclera. This sign indicates an inability of the digestive system to metabolize protein efficiently.

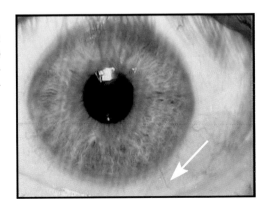

12. Chain of Pearls sign

This sign appears as a small vessel connecting several spots. It indicates a weakness in the walls of blood vessels resulting in a tendency to bruise or bleed upon injury.

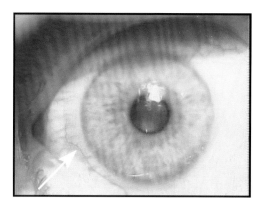

13. Pool vessels

These occur as a more serious progression of the Chain of Pearls sign where small pools of blood on a thin blood vessel occur. Indications include worsening in the integrity of the blood vessel walls and congestion with the possibility of a slow pulse. (bradycardia)

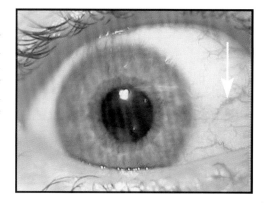

14. Melanin sign

Melanin deposits often occur in brown eyes due to heavy skin pigmentation as melanin overflows in the sclera next to the iris. If the deposit is located away from the iris in the sclera, it can indicate liver problems. In blue eyes it may indicate dysfunction of the pancreas or hardening of liver tissues.

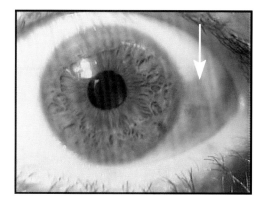

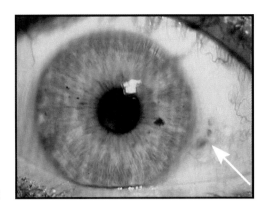

Melanin sign

15. Tape vessels

Tape vessels can occur as two or three parallel thick or thin vessels. They often indicate venous congestion, athero-sclerosis, hardening of the arteries or hemorrhoids.

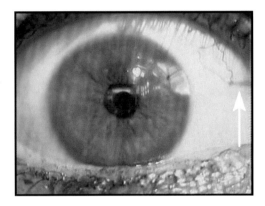

16. Glomeruli vessels

These vessels are rare to see but they indicate reduced peripheral blood flow due to constriction of capillaries owing to hormonal action or blockages. Renal problems such as kidney stones can occur.

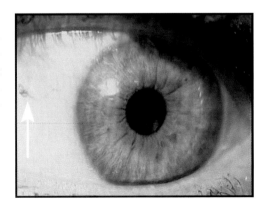

17. Pregnancy gender sign

As noted before, it is not possible to detect pregnancy in the iris because it is a natural process. There is a sign however, that has shown a certain amount of disputed accuracy after 28 weeks of pregnancy that may determine the sex of the child. This sign, a small blood vessel appearing in the right eye at 5 o'clock in the sclera opposite the uterus area, indicates a female child. The same sign in the same location opposite the ovary in the left eye indicates a male. I do not consider this sign to be very reliable but worth a try!

B. Non- Vascular Signs seen in the Sclera

1. Pinguecula

These are small, clear, yellow or orange fatty deposits often on the medial side in the sclera. Pinguecula can indicate a tendency toward gall bladder problems, poor fat metabolism, elevation of cholesterol and triglyceride levels and liver disease.

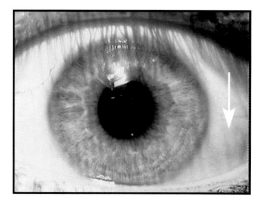

2. Pterygium

These appear as clear, white or yellow fatty deposits, usually vascular, that move over the iris border itself indicating liver problems.

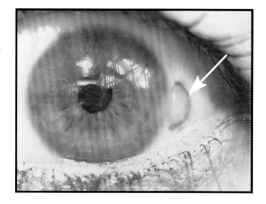

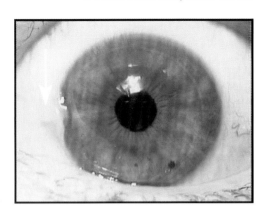

Pterygium

3. Fatty Liver sign

Seen as an accumulation of small, yellowish-brown fatty deposits on the medial side of the sclera, indicating the condition of fatty liver.

Chapter 18

The Brain, Psychological behavior and Iridology

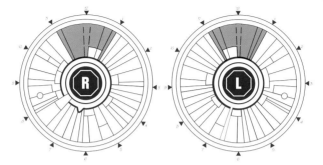

"The brain and psychology may be responsible for much more disease than we can ever imagine."

An understanding of physical indicators in the iris of the eye has led many iridologists to seek answers to mental or psychological factors through iris diagnosis examinations. The human brain, the least known organ of the body and the least known area in iridology, is still a mystery. The more we uncover, the more questions come up. Modern medicine tends to separate the physical from the psychological as separate entities and there are specialists for each of these fields. When I examine the eyes of patients who have psychological problems, I cannot help but make a close association between the physical weaknesses I see and the personality traits or psychological problems that I encounter. In holistic medicine we must take the entire individual's physical, mental, and spiritual health into consideration.

Who is to say that physical health status does not affect our attitudes, feelings, moods, and the way we interact with one another? Who is to say that anxiety, anger, hatred, jealousy or aggression are not spurred on by nutritional deficiencies in our body? Maybe if all of us received adequate nutrition and our bodies and brains received what they needed even when under stress, we would live in a much kinder and peaceful world without the threat of war. We all know how we feel when we eat poorly. We often suffer from depression, fatigue, or lack of ambition. Under these conditions we are like a time bomb when anything can set us off! Very soon negative feelings come into play, we become defensive, impatient, closed-minded and aggressive. We are ready to fight! It is no wonder that we often destroy marriages, friendships, and business relationships over the smallest, and most ridiculous things. When our physical bodies are not working properly there will always be psychological implications. The two are intertwined with one another. Studies with schizophrenics who were alcoholics indicated that they suffered a lack of Vitamin B as well as mineral deficiencies. Now is the fact that they were alcoholics the reason for the schizophrenia? We still do not know for sure but I can say that almost every patient I have had who suffered from severe psychological problems was much more capable of handling them, once his or her physical health status improved.

However, the opposite also applies. Not only does the physical affect the mental, but the psychological has significant influence upon our physical health as well. It seems that almost every cancer patient I have had, had endured a long or intense period of stress some time before the prognosis. The loss of a loved one, a divorce, loneliness, problems at work, or financial stress always carry with them an increased incidence of disease, lowered immunity, or just poor health in general. How many times have we witnessed the death of an older person and as early as a few months later their life-long partner died as well? When we lose our reason to live, our bodies rapidly deteriorate. Many alternative therapists concentrate on assisting their patients to let go of negative feelings that may be deeply imbedded. The consequent improvement in physical health is often amazing.

We cannot neglect the amount of stress we have today in our society. What we often forget is that we have the ability to control how this affects us. Stress places our bodies in an uncomfortable state of imbalance. Organs that normally function smoothly are suddenly placed under excessive strain, with an elevated need for nutrients. Our diets are often so inadequate that they do not supply our bodies with the required vitamins and minerals even under normal conditions. How then, can they function with the additional burden of excess stress? We need to put things into perspective. Why are we always in a hurry? Why do we skip meals during work? Why do we stay up all night and not enjoy regular quality sleep? Why do we wait until the weekend or until we go on holidays to finally relax? If the reason is that as human beings we have learned to be competitive in order to ensure our survival, then we are not being very practical. A hectic lifestyle where we neglect our health and allow stress to slowly undermine our bodies is not the answer. If we are interested in being a productive and efficient organism, which will not succumb to every infection or disease that comes along and which has the capacity for living to 150 years, we need to make positive lifestyle changes.

While I can appreciate that many serious mental problems stem from childhood and the effect of the environment around us as well as hereditary factors, we still have a greater chance of psychological improvement if our physical health receives assistance along with our mental health. People who are under a heavy psychological burden will eventually succumb to physical manifestations of disease.

In my study of iridology, the greatest incidence of psychological ill health has always been evident when one or more of the elimination organs were weak. These include the kidneys, liver, digestive system, lungs, lymphatic system, and skin. As we have discovered in a previous chapter, inadequate function in these organs or systems results in the accumulation of unwanted toxins in the body. One of the organs most rapidly affected by such toxins is the human brain.

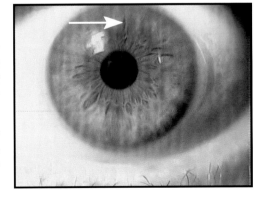

The effects of increased toxicity are seen as changes in color, flecks, lacunae, nerve rings or channels in the top area of the iris map called the **Brain Zone**.

This zone is located between 11 o'clock and 1 o'clock in both right and left irises and as mentioned before, it is an area that is still relatively unknown.

However, I have divided the brain zone into a number of different areas based on correlations between physical and psychological problems with what I had seen in this part of the iris. Physical effects are described first, followed by the many psychological implications of iris signs.

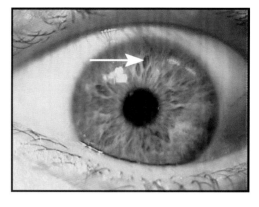

Right in the center of the brain zone we find the **Vitality-Fatigue** area, which represents the hypothalamus, the area of the brain which controls physical and mental energy levels and metabolism. Any unusual colors, lacunae, or markings in this area can point to physical changes in the hypothalamus as well as having corresponding psychological impli-

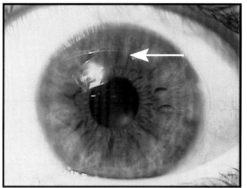

cations. If there are unusual white flecks or marks in this area, there is usually hyperactivity, often accompanied by headaches. If there are dark spots or markings they commonly indicate low energy levels.

Surrounding the Vitality-Fatigue area in the iris are centers for our **sensory and motor functions, learning centers, and logical thought processes.** When lacunae or radii solarii are found in this area the related functions can be weakened resulting in difficulties in learning, memory, sensory perception, motor control and reasoning.

The **Sleep Center** is also located in the brain zone and lesions in this area can affect our sleep and wake cycles, and quality of sleep.

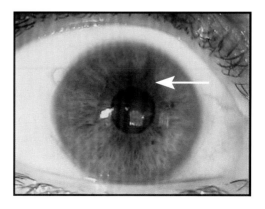

At 11 o'clock in the right iris and at 1 o'clock in the left iris we see the **Breathing Center.** This center represents the medulla, which controls respiratory rhythm. If dark signs like lacunae or radii solarii appear in this area they can represent conditions like asthma or bronchitis or other respiratory conditions.

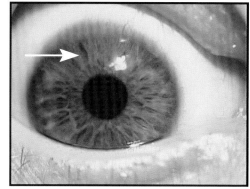

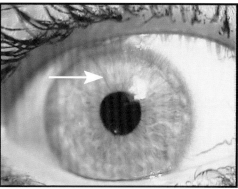

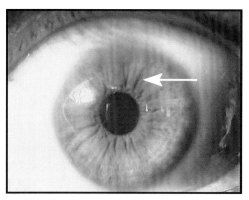

In the left iris only, next to the breathing center, is where the **Balance Center** of the body is located. White signs in this area usually indicate dizziness, and dark signs, although not always accurate can be sometimes seen in epilepsy or indicate inner ear problems with physical balance.

The **temple** is located next to the sleep center in both irises and unusual markings in this area are associated with headaches, migraines and sometimes tinnitus or ringing in the ears.

Psychological manifestations of clouds, radii solarii, lacunae, nerve rings, and arcus senilus are briefly discussed below.

It should be noted that these signs could also indicate physical disturbances in the brain along with the psychological.

1. Clouds in the periphery of the brain zone

Clouds in the outer ring of the iris in the brain zone indicate that the lymphatic system is congested and unable to efficiently cleanse the body of unwanted toxins, which have now accumulated in the tissues of the brain. Often there is heavy fatigue, depression, mood changes and feelings of anxiety. The clouds may range from white to yellow to brown, depending on kidney or liver involvement.

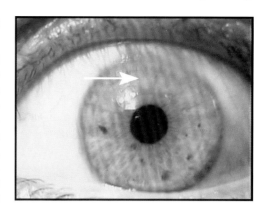

2. Radii solarii from the ruff zone through the vitality- fatigue zone

These are channels that range from white to dark which begin in the ruff zone and run upwards through the vitality- fatigue zone. Often the cause of this problem stems from a very toxic digestive system and Leaky Gut syndrome where unwanted substances are entering the blood through the intestinal walls and affecting other body tissues such as the brain. The vitality-fa-

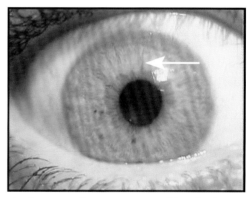

tigue zone is a very critical area in the brain that controls our energy and inspiration, as well as our emotional balance. When white channels are seen it often indicates hyperactive or extroverted behavior, while dark channels may indicate low vitality, depression, introverted behavior, pessimism, or paranoia depending on the severity of the sign.

3. Radii solarii through the balance center

In the left iris in the brain zone before 1 o'clock is the Balance Center. Radii solarii, lacunae, or flecks that are seen through this area affect our sense of emotional balance, intuition, and judgment. Commonly seen psychological behavior is insecurity, mood fluctuations, rash decision-making, stubbornness, and neuroses.

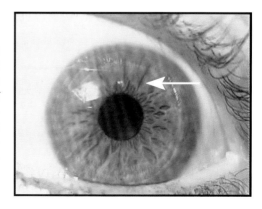

4. Lacunae in the brain zone

Any lacunae in the brain zone depending on whether it is acute or chronic can affect behavior. Generally the cause is inadequate blood flow to the area of the brain resulting in degeneration of tissue. Common problems include depression, anxiety, obsessive behavior, and negative thinking.

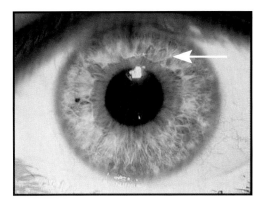

5. Nerve rings in the brain zone

As mentioned before, nerve rings result from chronic stress and can be seen in any part of the iris. When seen in the brain zone, they may indicate a tendency to suppress emotions and difficulties in expressing them.

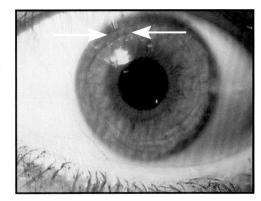

6. Arcus senilus

The arcus senilus, a white arc that is seen in the upper brain area indicates arteriosclerosis or hardening of the arteries due to fat and cholesterol deposits. People with this sign often suffer from senility, irrational behavior, depression, anxiety, or loss of memory.

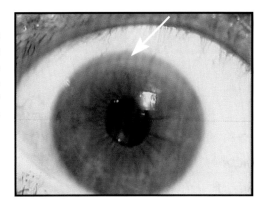

7. Drug spot accumulations

Some drugs have been found to accumulate in the body or brain tissue itself, leaving drug spots of a variety of colors in the brain area of the iris. Accumulation of drugs in the body may be due to a damaged liver or other elimination organs. A variety of psychological symptoms can sometimes be seen depending on the location of the spots and color.

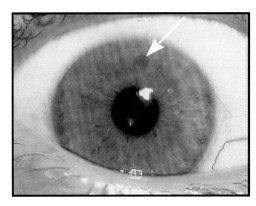

In a previous chapter we discussed the pupil and how it often reveals problems in our nervous system and spinal areas. A few cases that reveal psychological behavior are worth noting. See the chapter on the pupil for iris examples.

1. Size of pupil

People with very small pupils **(miosis)** are often seen to change behavior dramatically from one extreme to the other. They are often perfectionists, leaders in society, and very goal-oriented. They are often impatient with others and may sometimes forget about people due to their great drive and ambition.

Those with very large pupils **(mydriasis)** have a much softer personality, which is very sensitive and can feel stress quite easily. These people are usually friendly, approachable and interact well with people. They are often very intuitive but they can be taken advantage of, or misled.

When **anisocoria** is present (one pupil is dramatically larger than the other) it may signify a heavy psychological burden or in the condition known as **hippus** (pupils change rapidly in size), dramatic mood changes may be seen.

2. Ellipsoid pupils

Often depression and at times suicidal tendencies are seen with ellipsoid pupils.

3. Pupil Flattening

A superior flattening in the right eye often indicates serious depression, pessimism and negative thinking, and a false sense of reality. There were a few cases that I have seen where there had been a dramatic superior flattening and after questioning, the patient admitted to thoughts of, or attempts at suicide. A superior flattening in the left eye often indicates aggressive tendencies, an explosive temper, or violent behavior.

Finally, we must also take into account the role of genetic influence on our behavioral patterns. A number of genetic iris constitutions that we have previously mentioned have associated personality traits. Below are a few cases that are worth mentioning.

1. Neurolymphatic iris constitution

This genetic type as we have discussed before, indicates individuals who are very sensitive to stress and often find it difficult to overcome emotional traumas. They often suffer from anxiety, neuroses, fear, variable moods, and skepticism. Other characteristics include being very easily hurt in relationships, worrying unnecessarily over other people's problems and suffering nervous breakdowns under great stress.

2. Hematogenic iris constitution

Personality traits in the hematogenic constitution often include impulsive, or hyperactive behavior. These individuals are often overly emotional, easily excited, and quick-tempered.

3. Plethoric iris constitution

The Plethoric iris constitution often suffers from moody and irritable behavior with depression.

4. Hormonal iris constitution

Often depression or hyperactivity is seen.

5. Hydro-lymphatic iris constitution

Depression, mood changes, and impatient behavior are commonly seen.

Chapter 19

10 Incurable Diseases of Modern Civilization

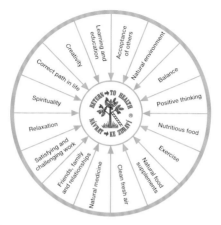

"We cannot gain health with our wealth, but through our behavior. Diet and lifestyle changes can produce what modern medicine calls, miracles."

As we have now covered the majority of iris signs, pupil signs, and sclera signs that we can see in the iris, I am sure you have come to appreciate the complexity of this new science of iridology. One general conclusion you may have come up with is that our society suffers from a lot of unnecessary disease. The cost of medical and hospital care for these sick people is astronomical. Health problems continue to rise. The rate of cancer and diabetes is climbing. What does this say about the way we approach our health? We leave it to the last possible minute and then we are paying for it, both physically and from our pockets in taxes. If we could change the way we approach health and look at it in terms of prevention rather than treatment, we would save money and gain valuable, healthy years to our lives. Although in certain cases these conditions may be genetically acquired, I believe that 90 percent of these diseases are due to improper diet and lifestyle decisions.

This chapter is about ten of the most commonly encountered problems that I see today for which modern medicine has no concrete cure, and how iridology can assist to uncover their causes.

1. Eczema
2. Irritable bowel syndrome
3. Migraine headaches
4. High blood pressure
5. Cancer
6. Asthma
7. Allergies
8. Pre-menstrual syndrome, irregular periods, menopausal symptoms
9. Osteoporosis
10. Arthritis

1. Eczema

Eczema is a skin condition commonly seen today in young children and adults. Often children as they say, grow out of the condition as they get older but in either case modern medicine does not really have a cure. External ointments like antibiotics or corticoids may cover up the problem initially, but the cause of the problem is left untreated. As we have learned, the skin is one of the detoxification organs in the body and chronic skin conditions are a sign that the body is finding it difficult to rid itself of toxins. Unnatural methods of treatment will force the elimination process backwards and this may later result in even more serious conditions. Ask yourselves, have you really treated the cause or just the symptoms of the disease?

The skin zone in the outer ring of the iris is a good indicator for the condition of the skin. Look for a darkening of the ciliary border indicating suppression of toxins in the skin. Next to the skin zone is the lymphatic and blood circulation. It works hand in hand with the skin. Often white or dirty yellow brown clouds in this area indicate that the lymphatic system is congested with undigested fats and toxins are getting into the blood.

Look to the digestive system for signs of the Leaky Gut syndrome or around the pupil border for absorption problems. What is the condition of the kidneys and the liver? Take a look at the sclera for signs of poor circulation.

As you see, the iris can give valuable clues as to what is really happening in the patient's body. Once these weak areas are treated, the body will have the ability to heal itself, to clear itself of its toxic load, and often these skin conditions clear up. I believe that the most effective ways are through vitamin and mineral therapy and changes in diet and lifestyle. Treatment may take as long as two years or more, depending on the severity.

2. Irritable Bowel Syndrome

This condition affects thousands of people and results in patients who suffer from very watery diarrhea and may have to go to toilet up to fifteen times a day. We have learned in the chapter on the Digestive system and the Leaky Gut syndrome, that the micro floral environment is vital to our well-being and health. Look for a history of antibiotic use or other drug use. Take a look at the condition of the digestive system, the acidity, and absorption capabilities. Look for nerve rings in the iris indicating sensitivity to stress. Take a look at the condition of the liver and gall bladder. Are there signs that indicate that bile flow is inadequate or may be of poor quality? This can affect the pH of the intestines and cleansing of the digestive system. Is the pancreas supplying enough digestive enzymes? Worsening of this condition can lead to more serious chronic problems such as Colitis, or Crohn's syndrome. Are there any allergies? Does the genetic iris constitution indicate predisposition to certain problems? The iridologist must search for signs in the entire body to find what really is causing this problem. As every patient is unique, each must be looked at individually.

3. Migraine Headaches

The number of pharmaceutical preparations for headaches and migraines is a sign of the prevalence of this painful health problem in our society today.

What causes migraines? Nobody really knows the answer. There are drugs that can assist and in some cases people cannot live a normal life without them, but do we really want to be taking a pill every single time we have a headache? Wouldn't it be better to find the cause of the problem?

There may be many reasons why a migraine headache occurs. In my iris studies I have found several causes. The most frequent sign I see is a general toxic overload of the body, which can often be seen in the head or brain zone. Each of the detoxification organs must be looked at individually for signs of weakness. This includes the kidneys, as their insufficiency can increase the toxic load in the body and head area, as well as create edema and cause pressure in the head. The liver, skin, lymphatic system, and digestive system, need to be functioning at full capacity. Look for signs of stress and type of iris constitution for assistance in uncovering causes. The Neuro-Lymphatic iris constitution often suffers from migraines due to stress. Look for allergies. Often foods like chocolate, tomatoes, coffee, red wine, cheese, artificial sweeteners, and monosodium glutamate have been linked to migraine headaches. What is the condition of the circulatory system? Is there arteriosclerosis? Is the respiratory system providing enough oxygen to the tissues? Is the blood sugar fluctuating? Is there flattening on the pupil indicating neck or cervical spine problems? Any one of these conditions can result in migraine headaches.

4. High Blood Pressure

We do not really know why some people get high blood pressure. Usually this occurs as we age but its incidence has been linked to heart disease, heart attacks, strokes, and kidney problems. When the blood pressure is too high, blood vessels or organs can be damaged. The combination of the pressures of all the blood vessels in the body, the veins, arteries, and capillaries must be in perfect balance in order that every cell of the body receives oxygen and nutrients. The heart must also be strong and in perfect rhythm to provide the correct amount of cardiac output with each beat. It must also be in excellent condition to allow for the resting phase and the filling of the heart chambers in preparation for the pumping of the blood.

Stress plays a big part especially in the top systolic number of the blood pressure reading. The quality of the blood and the components in the blood are also important in blood pressure. Our excessive intake of salt is a factor in hypertension or high blood pressure as well.

It is important to look in the iris and sclera at the condition of the blood vessels. Have they lost their elasticity or flexibility? Are there conditions indicating hemorrhoids or varicose veins? What is the condition of the kidneys and their ability to control water and salt balance in the body? Is the patient under stress? Are there signs of high cholesterol, atherosclerosis, or arteriosclerosis? Check the liver as it produces plasma proteins that affect the composition of the blood. Remember to always look at the body holistically, as an integrated system.

5. Cancer

Cancer is a major cause of death in our society today. The incidence of cancer is rising despite modern technology and its efforts to find a drug cure for this disease. Why can we not find a cure for cancer? There have been so many links to cancer including certain carcinogenic foods, smoking, sunshine, chemicals and every day we hear of something else that causes cancer. What really causes our cells in the body to change and instead of helping us, begin to fight against us? No one knows exactly. Modern medicine is left with only a few alternatives, surgical operations to remove the tumor, radiation, and chemotherapy. These are all very drastic measures. Often after a cancer operation, metastasis occurs. Why? It's because any operation that we undertake, results in stress to our body, and lowered immunity. The body is now in a weakened state. Do we really want to radiate our bodies and pump in high concentrations of drugs in order to kill the cancer cells as well as our healthy cells? Is this what our body needs? Extra toxicity? Several years ago, I watched this process with my mother who after eight years died of ovarian cancer. The radiation treatment in the initial stage caused problems five years later in her digestive system and she had to undergo an ileostomy and colostomy. Three six- month sessions of chemotherapy not only resulted in loss of hair but in excessive vomiting, pain and lowered immunity. No one can convince me that this is what our body needs to heal itself from cancer. Perhaps these methods can save some lives in emergency situations, but they certainly should not be the ultimate solutions for the cure of cancer in the future.

I believe that cancer is an autoimmune disease where the cells change due to chronic stress or inflammation for long periods of time. This can be applied to excessive sunlight or sunburn that can cause chronic skin inflammation and cause skin cancer. Smoking creates chronic inflammation in the lungs and increases the incidence of lung cancer. Chronic constipation and bowel problems are associated with bowel cancers. Whether we get cancer or not, depends on the strength of our genetic constitution as well as our ability to eliminate toxins and wastes from our bodies. If we suppress our disease with drugs, the symptoms can go away but the core of the problem is left untreated. In time, the condition reaches a chronic and then degenerative stage where there is possibility of the cells mutating or changing. Every cancer patient that I have had has shown a high level of toxicity in the body.

Take a good look, especially at the iris for toxic signs in the digestive system and radii solarii, signs of liver or kidney weakness, and lung, lymphatic, or skin congestion. Dark deep lacunae indicate degenerate conditions that can lead to tumor or cancer formation. All the elimination or detoxification channels need to be working effectively, for all waste products to clear the body. When the body is toxic, regeneration is slow and the immune system is slow to respond. Look for inflammation signs around organs, indicating acute signals and do not neglect signs of stress, like nerve rings. Most cancer patients I speak with have had a long period of stress prior to their diagnosis. The body needs adequate

ingestion: nutrients including high quality foods, megavitamin therapy, and oxygen, efficient **digestion** and **absorption**, **circulation** to transport these nutrients and to clear toxins, **utilization** of nutrients that are brought to the cells, and the ability to eliminate waste products for **detoxification** of the body. These, as outlined in a previous chapter, are the essential processes of life. The management of cancer or any other disease must always take these into consideration.

6. Asthma

Asthma is another disease that I frequently encounter in practice. The number of asthma sufferers is very high, especially in Australia where I used to live.

This is still a condition for which there is no cure. Every year, many people die of asthma attacks. Many children as well as adults suffer from this respiratory condition, which can be brought on by allergies, exercise, stress, or other causes.

Generally bronchial dilating drugs are used to relieve asthma but the side effects of constant chemical stimulation of the bronchial passages to dilate, are not very positive and again they do not address the cause of the problem.

If a child or adult suffers from asthma they should not be consuming milk products as they are very mucous forming and many people are allergic to the lactose in milk or milk products. What many parents of asthmatic children worry about when milk products are removed from their child's diet, is where they will get their calcium. Only about ten percent of the calcium phosphate in milk is absorbable, while calcium carbonate in green leafy vegetables, fish, almonds, and sesame seeds, has a much higher absorption rate and is a source of better- quality calcium in the diet. If there is too much mucus in the breathing passages, then irritants like dust or other pollutants can get lodged, and bring on asthma as well.

When examining the iris, look for weakness signs or inflammation signs in the bronchi, bronchioles, and lungs. Look for allergy signs in the sclera. The condition of the bowel can also indicate causes of asthma as the Leaky Gut syndrome generates a large amount of free radicals that form lipid peroxides, which can cause irritation of the mucous membranes. Treatment often involves repairing the lining of the intestinal walls and improving the favorable bacteria in the intestines. Look for signs of stress as well as flattening on the pupil, which can indicate nervous system causes of respiratory problems. The breathing center in the brain zone can also point to asthma or respiratory problems.

7. Allergies

The incidence and the number of allergies that exist today seem to be rapidly growing. Hay fever, dust, pollens, and allergies to a variety of foods plague a high percent of the population. Children often suffer a host of allergic symptoms like runny nose, itchy and swollen eyes, sneezing, and skin rashes.

While allergy tests such as the pinprick skin tests may isolate an allergy to a certain substance, the cause of allergies is still virtually unknown.

With the increased ingestion of chemically prepared foods, smog and pollutants in the air, as well as the thousands of drugs that are available to treat the many conditions we have, it is no wonder that our society is suffering from allergies. I believe that allergies are the body's reaction or attempt to rid it of toxic substances. I do not believe that any person should be allergic to a natural food substance. Allergies to foods may initially start from the Leaky Gut syndrome, where larger food molecules begin to leak through the intestinal wall into the bloodstream. The immune system reacts as if it were a foreign substance and an allergy may develop. Treatment of the Leaky Gut syndrome often improves this condition. I have seen this in practice and with time the patient was able to consume the food to which he had previously been allergic.

Allergy signs can be seen in the sclera. Look for signs especially in the digestive system as well as congestion in the skin and lymphatic system and inflammation signs in the lungs or bronchial passages. Pay attention to weakness signs in any of the detoxification organs.

8. Pre-menstrual syndrome, Irregular periods, Menopause symptoms

It seems that every other female I see, suffers from menstrual pain, difficulties, or irregular periods. There is also an increasing amount of fertility problems. A normal period should last about three days but most people accept 5 or 7 days as normal. As mentioned before, the use of oral contraceptives and hormone replacement therapies has created chaos in the hormonal system of the body. With oral contraceptives there is a greater tendency toward heart disease and liver problems while the incidence of breast and uterine cancer has increased with the use of hormone replacement therapy. It is my belief that their use has contributed to many problems we have today. The body needs to find its own hormonal balance through natural means. Often the pituitary gland and adrenal gland are weakened and there is an imbalance in the hormones that are secreted. This can result in heavy, painful, or delayed periods. In order to have a 28 -day cycle, the pituitary gland and adrenal gland must be in balance. Often, if menstrual problems are not corrected at an early age, or symptoms are suppressed as in oral contraceptive use, difficulties can occur later in menopause. High blood sugar or fluctuating blood sugar levels can also affect the hormonal system and stress can exhaust the adrenal glands. Vitamin and mineral therapy along with a correct diet often helps to correct these problems within a period of several months.

Look for weakness signs in the pituitary and adrenal glands in the iris, especially radii solarii, signs of stress as in nerve rings, inflammation signs in the uterus or ovaries, drug spots throughout the iris or liver problems.

Deficiencies in digestion and absorption can often be seen in the stomach and intestinal rings as well as around the pupil border. Look also for signs of blood sugar fluctuations.

9. Osteoporosis

Osteoporosis has been given much media attention in recent years especially as a problem in post-menopausal women. Osteoporosis is caused by a loss of calcium from the bones, leading to bone demineralization and weakness. This disease accounts for a high incidence of hip and bone fractures in the elderly. Exercise that involves weight bearing activities as well as a sound nutritional program can improve bone density and strength and slow down the process of osteoporosis.

An analysis of the iris often indicates weakness signs in the digestive system where the stomach often lacks hydrochloric acid so that protein digestion is limited. This indicates an accumulation of acid-forming bacteria in the intestines. A healthy digestive system will ensure that calcium and other essential minerals and vitamins needed for bone formation are adequately absorbed into the blood system. Look for signs in the endocrine glands indicating hormonal imbalance, as well as signs in the liver. A notched pupil border also indicates weakness in the joints and bones. Look also at possible circulation problems like varicose veins or weakness in blood vessels, seen in the sclera.

10. Arthritis

Arthritis is an inflammation of the joints that affects many individuals, especially the elderly. The synovial fluid, that is the fluid within the joints becomes too watery and loses its lubricating nature. While there are many preparations on the market for arthritis including creams and ointments, as well as anti-inflammatory drugs, they only serve to reduce some of the painful symptoms but again do not address the cause. Often this can be traced back to the digestive system. Excessive growth of harmful bacteria like Candida albicans and E.coli as well as others in the intestines can form an acidic environment and cause damage to the intestinal walls as in the Leaky Gut syndrome. The free radicals that are generated once in the bloodstream can form lipid peroxides, which destroy tissue cells, and can affect the joints and synovial fluid. The liver also is affected, as it must neutralize the extra lactic acid in the urea cycle.

Signs in the iris indicating causes of arthritis often include the Leaky Gut syndrome or weakness signs in the digestive system, and weaknesses in the liver sector or toxic brown spots throughout the iris. Often in blue eyes, the effects of over acidity can be seen dramatically in white inflammation signs covering almost the entire iris. Blue eye genetic iris types, especially the lymphatic constitutions have an increased predisposition to arthritis.

Chapter 20
Healing Methods and Iridology

Healing lines

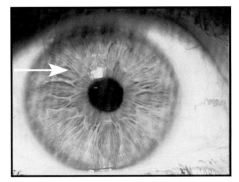

"It is nice to know the name of your disease but much nicer to know a method to cure it."

A diagnostic method is only as good as its ability to find a method to cure the diagnosed problems. What good is it if we find out everything that is wrong with us but there is no prescribed treatment? We had seen that there are many diseases that are incurable but iridology has been able to shed some light on what may be possible causes. So much time is taken forcing the patient through a variety of classical tests only to discover that there is only a minimum that can be done for treatment. There are many alternative medicine methods that deal with disease in a natural way, including herbal medicine, homeopathy, and a variety of body therapies but I will discuss the two that are very close to my heart; **Nutritional therapy** and **Bowen pressure therapy**. I have chosen these healing methods because I had found them particularly beneficial in that they work hand in hand with the science of iridology, as they take the individual patient into consideration and provide a holistic approach.

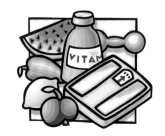

Nutritional Therapy

What is nutritional therapy?

Our bodies can be described as large, complex, chemical factories. They utilize our ingested nutrients to build, repair, and regenerate all the tissues in the body. Without these nutrients, cells will stop functioning and die. The organs and systems in our body then break down and allow disease to enter. Without the essential life process of ingestion we have no digestion, absorption, circulation, utilization, and detoxification. In every nutritional program there must be a solid foundation of healthy eating habits. However, curing a disease often involves much more than just diet alone. Nutritional therapy consists of a program tailor-made for the individual patient, which includes diet and lifestyle changes and nutritional supplements to maintain health and regenerate diseased tissue.

Why can't we get everything from food?

Achieving our nutritional daily requirement solely from food would be possible in an ideal world with no smog, pollution, or stress, and fresh food without preservatives or chemical additives. This is not to say, it is impossible in modern times, but it is much more difficult and probably the greatest challenge we face today.

In the real world we consume thousands of different chemicals in foods, including coloring agents, preservatives, and other additives. Our fruits and vegetables are grown in soil that is not always free of contaminants, not to mention the loss of valuable vitamins through storage and transportation. Due to competition as well as our insistent demand for perfect- looking foods, manufacturers are spraying vegetables and fruit with harmful chemicals, scientists are busy genetically changing our foods, and preservatives and colors are being added to most of them. In summary, the quality of our food supply is in danger if we continue on this path. It is affecting the health of our bodies and increasing the toxic load on our detoxification organs. If the human race does not destroy itself through world wars, it may do so by poisoning its own food supply.

In our stressful lives we often choose to buy more fast foods, and processed foods with longer expiry dates. We do not take the time to fix a fresh, healthy meal. We violate the laws that nature has handed down to us. Is it possible to maintain our health in such a hectic and chaotic lifestyle?

Why do we need extra vitamins and supplements?

The majority of us have diets that are lacking in quality nutrients, not only because we eat poorly but also because the foods we eat lack many nutrients. Each one of us, as we have learned, is born with certain genetic traits and so we start our lives with some organs weaker than others. This is what we mean by our genetic iris constitution. As a result of iris examination we can diagnose what problems there are and compensate for our weaknesses. By providing the body with specifically tailored extra nutrients that can regenerate and strengthen the weaker organs, we can prevent the occurrence of disease in the future. Nutrition for genetic iris constitutions is dealt with in much greater detail in my book, "The Eye for an Eye diet."

Does Nutritional Therapy work?

I have used nutritional therapy for many years based on what I had seen in the iris. Not only does it allow for natural regeneration of organs and detoxification of the body but it can also be seen as healing signs in the iris. Remember the healing crisis. In order to really achieve true health, we must allow the body to pass through periods where some of our suppressed diseases come to the surface as in the acute stage. Only when our body clears itself of all toxins, will our health have a chance to improve. Nutritional therapy accelerates the process and allows the body to regenerate much faster and to pass through several healing crises so that the patient can once again return to health. Nutritional therapy does not mask the symptoms of disease but provides the building blocks so that the body can heal itself. Along with the diagnostic tool of iridology, nutritional therapy provides an invaluable method for preventing and curing many of the diseases that plague modern society.

Bowen Pressure Therapy

When I lived in Australia, I was very fortunate to come across a wonderful therapeutic technique called the Bowen Method. During my time there I had the opportunity to study this technique with some of the pioneers of a method that today is taught in over 25 countries around the world. Today, this technique remains as mysterious as its founder, Mr. Tom Bowen who according to some accounts said that he had received the gift from God. After serving in World War 2, Tom Bowen became interested in ways to relieve human suffering and developed the technique without any previous training in health care. By 1975 Mr. Bowen was treating over 13.000 patients per year and people would literally line up at his door.

After his death in 1986, the technique began to be taught in Australia by a couple, the Rentsches, who had studied with Mr. Bowen and documented his work. Soon it was being taught all over Australia, New Zealand, North America, the United Kingdom, and Europe.

What is Bowen Pressure Therapy?

Bowen Pressure Therapy is a dynamic system of muscle and connective tissue massage that is revolutionizing health care worldwide. For over 40 years it has been successfully used to assist thousands of people who suffer from a variety of diseases. This technique has amazed therapists and doctors of all disciplines yet no one really knows exactly how it works. Yes, even today it remains a mystery and thousands of Bowen therapists would love to ask Mr. Bowen himself, if he were alive, how and why this technique works so effectively.

What seems to surprise many people is the fact that the Bowen method uses only gentle moves, yet strong amazing effects are regularly both seen and felt. People with severe back or neck pain often get relief after only 3 sessions, migraine headaches subside, and ankle, shoulder, and knee problems improve. There have even been cases where scoliosis or severe back curvatures actually straightened after this technique had been administered.

The Bowen method has been so successful in Australia that some veterinarians have adapted the method and now certain techniques are being used on racing horses and dogs with great success.

For what conditions can the Bowen method be used?

It has been used for conditions as diverse as tinnitus, allergies, asthma, bladder infections, high or low blood pressure, depression and psychological problems, eczema, gall bladder pain, kidney problems, and problems with menstruation.

The Bowen method is not acupressure or acupuncture but it corresponds to some similar locations but without needles or electronic equipment. It is safe to use on anyone from neonates to the aged and produces lasting relief from pain and discomfort.

After using this technique now for several years, I have been able to assist hundreds of clients with a variety of problems. I have successfully dealt with problems such as ringing in the ears or tinnitus, low immunity, malfunction of kidneys, migraines, stress and psychological problems, and joint and neck pain. Arthritic pain has been relieved, as well as pain from urinary bladder infections. I have been able to see marked improvement in asthma and breathing difficulties. Other results of the Bowen method include a decrease in high blood pressure, as well as many other positive improvements. Almost everyone receives some benefit from the Bowen method.

What separates the Bowen method of pressure therapy from other types of massage?

I believe the Bowen method works by balancing the body, so that it can once again allow itself to heal. It removes any blocks in the body that result from improper posture, lack of exercise, or injury and resets the whole body and its systems. The Bowen method utilizes the principle of positive and negative moves. Generally, the skin where the move is made is pulled back taut in a negative direction and then the move is made in the opposite direction over muscles, nerves, and ligaments. Those moves send an intricate message to the brain to initiate a series of reactions that provide muscle release reducing any tension in the area. While one move can have a beneficial effect, the whole series of moves in correct sequence, definitely has the greatest effect on the body.

I often compare our body to a guitar or a musical instrument that is constantly in need of tuning. Every day we abuse our bodies. We sleep on poor mattresses with too many pillows so that our spine is not resting in its natural state. We exercise improperly, we run with poor running shoes that do not absorb the shock, we lift objects without bending our knees or keeping a straight back, we reach for things in the back of the car when we are in the drivers seat, we carry bags on usually only one shoulder which places strain on one side of the body, plus a number of other activities which create an imbalance in our vertebral column. That imbalance places our muscular system on guard, which attempts to contract those muscles on one side of the body, to compensate for the shifts in our center of gravity.

Once those muscles are in a defense mode they maintain the new center of gravity and we then find that muscle tension is not properly in balance as one side has greater tension than the other. Our body then moves from its natural state of equilibrium and flexibility is reduced, our range of motion is reduced and so on.

As a result, problems like migraines, neck and back pain or joint problems may develop. Often in practice, I see many clients who have one leg longer than the other. Generally, that is not due to genetic defects, but to the pelvis being uneven with one side being higher than the other. Very often, after the Bowen method, that imbalance is rectified and the pelvis corrects itself.

Cysts and edema often improve with the Bowen method. I believe this is due to the stimulation of the body's cleansing organs like the kidneys as well as the drainage of the lymphatic system, which improves the body's immunity.

Pregnant mothers can get great relief from the Bowen method by its ability to relieve lower back pain while changes in the mother's body occur.

People under severe stress, anxiety, or depression often improve, and they begin to see problems in a different light as they receive physical and psychological relief from the Bowen method. I am not saying that this occurs in every case but clients often say that they feel like a weight has been lifted off them, that they have more energy and can focus better on the activities in their lives.

In almost every case of extreme migraine or head pain, I have seen relief or at least partial relief for up to six months after only a few sessions with the Bowen method. It greatly relieves a problem that plagues many people.

For the client, the Bowen method is virtually pain-free and non-invasive, and there is no need to remove clothing for the procedures. In most cases, the client comes in for three 30- minute sessions, which have been spaced five to ten days apart. In about 20 percent of cases, there may be a feeling of fatigue or nausea for the first few days after the application, so the client is encouraged to rest and to abstain from vigorous activity during that time. Generally, that feeling passes and is usually replaced with a greater sense of well-being.

For the Bowen Method to be completely effective, it is important not to undergo any manipulative therapy including classical massage four days before, and up to five days after, your Bowen therapy sessions. It should be strongly stressed that it is crucial for the client to drink a lot of water, a minimum of two liters a day as this method often creates a large amount of detoxification in the body, allowing the kidneys and detoxification organs to cleanse it of additional waste products.

Clients are also discouraged from bathing in very hot water or very cold water because this could reduce the effect of the technique as the Bowen method involves energy flow through the meridians of the body.

I recommend this technique to anyone who is suffering from any kind of chronic pain, suffering a lot of stress, or to those who are constantly feeling tired and lack energy. You will be pleasantly surprised at the effects of the Bowen method.

In my opinion, the Bowen method has produced some astounding results and doctors in Australia are currently researching how and why it works. Perhaps it is not so important to scientifically rationalize Mr. Tom Bowen's work. What is more important is to take advantage of its positive benefits that have helped thousands of people around the world. The Bowen method is a unique Australian method that stimulates the body to heal itself.

Chapter 21

Case Studies in Iridology

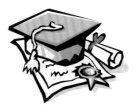

"Knowledge through experience is the greatest teacher."

The study of iridology in school certainly gave me the groundwork and foundation in the field, but it was through actual practice that I have gained invaluable experience. By analyzing thousands and thousands of irises over the years and speaking to thousands of patients with problems ranging from headaches to cancer, epilepsy to diabetes, I have acquired an invaluable resource of data and experience. In some cases it confirmed what I had learned in school, but in other cases it cast new light on and provided insights onto signs and conditions in the iris that I had never seen before. One thing that I have learned to appreciate is that iridology does not diagnose disease. Iridology diagnoses the causes of disease by revealing which organs and systems are weak or degenerating.

The science of iridology is still in infancy. I continue to see new signs or perhaps once in a while even an iris type that I have never encountered. I believe we have only touched the tip of the iceberg. That is the beauty of iridology. One cannot help but be constantly reminded that each one of us is different.

The following nine case studies are taken from actual patient files.

Case 1. Female, Age 20

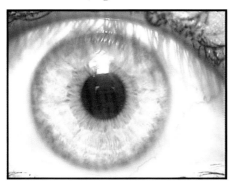

Right Eye

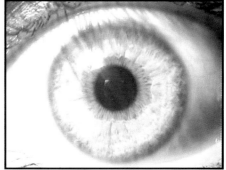

Left Eye

Main complaints: headaches, skin problems, recurrent bladder infections, constant fatigue

Iris Signs – Kidney Lymphatic iris constitution
– Degeneration of joints seen around pupil border
– Meander vessel in sclera indicates weakness in veins, and predisposition to varicose veins
– Darkened ruff zone
– Weakness signs through both kidney zones
– Nerve rings indicating high sensitivity to stress
– Darkened ciliary border
– Yellow color around ruff border indicating kidney involvement
– White color indicating over-acidic body fluids and tissues
– Clouds indicating congestion in the lymphatic system
– Acute sign in urinary bladder area
– Radii solarii running through adrenal gland in left iris
– Lesion in cervical spine area left iris and right neck
– Bronchial passages show weakness signs
– Uterus weakness in right iris

Comments:

This type of iris usually suffers from kidney problems, which often worsen with time. This may cause the over acidity of the body tissues often leading to arthritis and degeneration of the joints. Poor kidneys can bring on headaches and fatigue as toxins stay in the body too long and are often associated with bladder infections. The weakness signs in the cervical spine and neck may also be the cause of headaches. The darkened ciliary border indicates skin problems probably caused by a sluggish and congested lymphatic system due to undigested fats in the intestines. The effects of a toxic environment in the intestines is seen as radii solarii have formed, indicating that toxicity is spreading to other tissues of the body. This patient is under a fair amount of stress, which is affecting body organs.

Case 2. Male Age 55

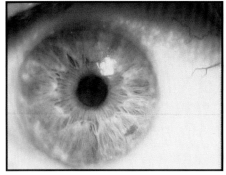
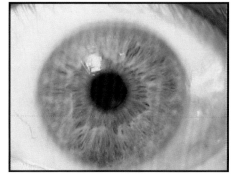

Right Eye   Left Eye

Main complaints: constipation, gall bladder pain, backache, breathing difficulties

Iris signs – Lymphatic Hypo-active iris constitution
– Toxic appearance
– Lateral pupil flattening
– Congested lymphatic system
– Weak right kidney
– Lacunae in gall bladder region
– Dark absorption ring
– Fork vessel and meander vessel in sclera
– Liver weakness signs
– Lacunae in breathing center

Comments:

This iris constitution has difficulty in removal of toxins from the body. The patient has a very toxic eye, congested lymphatic system, weaknesses in the liver and gall bladder with possible stone formation. The pupil flattening and lacunae in the breathing center indicate problems with respiration. The ability to absorb nutrients is low due to an over acid environment in the small intestines. Blood vessel signs in the sclera indicate a good chance of hemorrhoids or varicose veins.

Case 3. Female Age 24

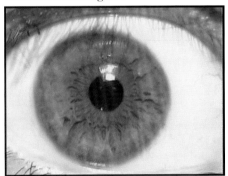 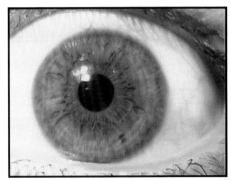

Right Eye   Left Eye

Main complaints: digestive problems, dizzy spells, hormonal problems, acne

Iris signs – Hematogenic iris constitution
– Nerve rings
– Darkening of the ciliary border
– Lacunae in pancreas, gall bladder, and heart zone areas
– Weakness signs in balance center
– Radii solarii in head area
– Uterus, and ovary signs
– Lower back weakness

    – Adrenal gland exhaustion
    – Liver spots

Comments:

This patient has a number of weaknesses seen as lacunae throughout parts of the iris. The digestive problems are probably due to bile flow from the gall bladder or insufficient digestive enzymes from the pancreas. The left and right side of the heart show weakness and potential for problems. A very sensitive nervous system where stress has exhausted the adrenal glands can lead to hormonal problems and fluctuations in blood sugar.

Radii solarii in the head area through the balance center indicate the possible cause of the dizzy spells. The darkened ciliary border indicates inability of the skin to eliminate toxins.

Case 4. Female Age 50

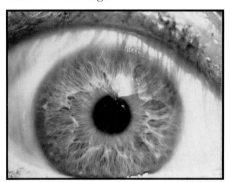 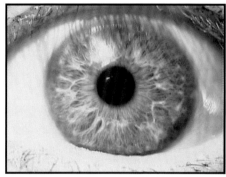

Right Eye   Left Eye

Main complaints: Diabetes, psoriasis, high blood pressure, overweight

Iris Signs – Lymphatic Hypo-active iris constitution
            – Dirty stomach ring
            – Ballooned bowel
            – Inflammation signs around autonomic nervous system
            – Lacunae in pancreas areas
            – Right adrenal gland weakness
            – Separation of fibers in thyroid areas and misty orange-yellow pigment
            – Right kidney weakness
            – Gall bladder
            – Inflammation signs in urinary bladder
            – Lacunae in uterus area

Comments:

The under-acid stomach and ballooned bowel indicate bacterial growth in the small intestine and loss of tone in the bowels resulting in reduced peristalsis. Pancreas and adrenal weakness has contributed to poor blood sugar control in the body. The under-active thyroid may be responsible for weight gain. Kidney weakness may be the cause of the high blood pressure and poor skin condition as well as poor elimination from the bowel. Acute signs in the gallbladder area indicate possibility of stones and reduction of bile flow to the duodenum, which will affect digestion.

Case 5. Female Age 59

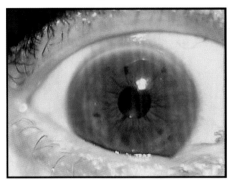 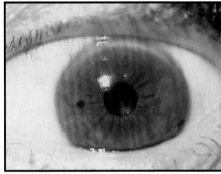

Right Eye   Left Eye

Main complaints: headache, poor memory, varicose veins, and high blood cholesterol

Iris signs – Hematogenic iris constitution
- Arcus senilus
- Liver spots
- Radii solarii
- Meander vessel in sclera
- Leaky Gut syndrome
- Cataract formation seen in pupil
- Nerve rings
- Pupil flattening

Comments:

This patient is suffering from a hardening of the arteries, which is affecting the brain as seen in the arcus senilus - white cap in the head area. Liver spots indicate the effects of drug accumulation in the body and the weakening of the liver. This may affect cholesterol levels in the blood and contribute to the arteriosclerosis. The intestinal zone is very toxic and there is evidence of the Leaky Gut syndrome, which is affecting digestion and ab-sorption. The appearance of radii solarii is indication that toxins are permeating through the intestinal wall and affecting other organs and tissues. Often hormonal problems can occur. Poor circulation in the form of weakened veins is seen by the appearance of vari-cose veins. There is evidence of many years of bad nutrition and a high cholesterol and fat diet.

Case 6. Male Age 58

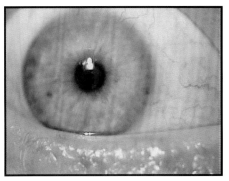 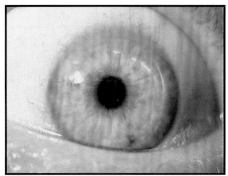

Right Eye   Left Eye

Main complaints: arthritis, pain in joints, back pain, fatigue, heartburn

Iris signs – Hydro-lymphatic iris constitution
– White over-acid appearance
– Nerve rings
– Liver spots
– Radii solarii
– Over-acid stomach ring
– Darkening of ciliary border
– Lymphatic clouds
– Absorption ring
– Weakness signs in prostate gland, upper left lung
– Inflammation signs on ruff zone border
– Radii solarii running up through vitality-fatigue zone
– Pupil flattening
– Blue along iris-sclera border

Comments:

This patient is displaying signs that his body is extremely over-acidic and white inflammation signs indicating an acute condition. The intestines are producing unfavorable bacteria, which are generating free radicals through the Leaky Gut syndrome and these are now affecting the joints and causing arthritis. This is indicated in the appearance of radii solarii and the poor absorptive ability seen in the absorption ring. There is inflammation of the nerves and flattening on the pupil border indicating possible pain and degeneration of the skeletal system. Breathing problems may be seen due to weaknesses in the lungs, and a lack of oxygen to the tissues indicated by a bluish ring around the iris next to the sclera. This lack of oxygen is affecting the brain and depleting energy levels as seen through weakness signs in the vitality-fatigue zone.

Case 7. Child male Age 8

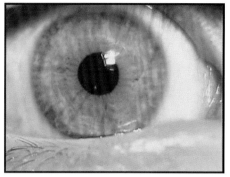 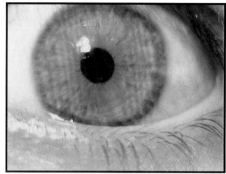

Right Eye   Left Eye

Main complaints: hyperactive, chronic sore throat, flu, colds, eczema

Iris signs   – Pancreatic colors
            – Right kidney weakness
            – Lymphatic clouds
            – Darkened ciliary border
            – Nerve rings
            – Open lacunae in left and right heart areas
            – Weakness signs in bronchial tubes
            – Separation in fibers in pancreas areas in left iris
            – Adrenal gland lacunae in right iris
            – Radii solarii in right iris

Comments:

This young child is already showing the beginning of some serious health problems. The predominance of orange color indicating pancreas involvement is confirmed with weakness signs in the pancreas areas in the left iris. This may cause blood sugar fluctuations and/or lack of pancreatic enzymes, which may explain the hyperactive behavior. Nerve rings indicate tension in the nervous system, which have affected the adrenal gland, which again can affect the blood sugar. The lymphatic circulation is showing extensive congestion and the skin zone is darkened indicating poor elimination of toxins, leading to the skin problems and lowered immunity. The right kidney weakness is also contributing to poor elimination of waste products. Bronchial tubes are showing inflammation signs and congestion leading to excessive mucus production and greater chance of bacterial or viral infections.

There are inherent weaknesses in the left and right side of the heart. Overgrowth of harmful bacteria in the intestines is probably due to repeated bouts of antibiotics.

Case 8. Female Age 32

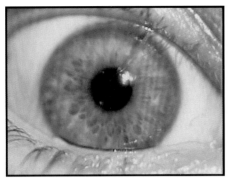 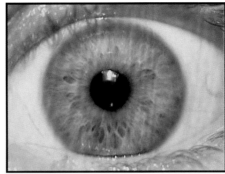

Right Eye   Left Eye

Main complaints: irregular periods, premenstrual syndrome, problems with sleep, frequent stomach upset

Iris signs – Hormonal iris constitution
– Multiple lacunae in glandular areas including pancreas, adrenal, thyroid, and pituitary
– Over-acid stomach ring
– Ballooned bowel
– Kidney weakness
– Signs in urinary bladder
– Radii solarii through pineal gland and sleep zone

Comments:

This type of iris is prone to problems with the hormonal system. Signs in the pancreas and adrenal glands can lead to blood sugar fluctuations. The thyroid shows weakness which can affect the heart as tachycardia and influence weight. The imbalance of hormones from the pituitary gland and the adrenal gland is most probably the cause of the irregular periods. There is a loss of tone in the bowel and over-acidity in the stomach, which can lead to constipation and ulcer formation. The weakness in the kidneys is also contributing to the over-acidity of the tissues, poor elimination of waste and subsequent infections of the urinary bladder. Toxicity is affecting the brain and the pineal gland and disturbing sleep patterns.

Case 9. Female Age 40

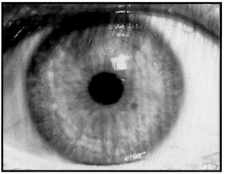 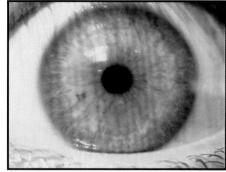

Right Eye   Left Eye

Main complaints: low immunity, chronic fatigue, ringing in ears (tinnitus), leg pain

Iris signs – Very toxic eye, drug accumulation
– Nerve rings in area of ovary, bladder, adrenal gland, and kidney
– Toxic lymphatic clouds
– Pancreatic and kidney colors
– Over-acidity of the tissues
– Toxic clouds over ear zone in right iris
– Weakness signs in legs
– Inferior pupil flattening in left iris

Comments:

These dramatic colors are often due to drug accumulation in the lymphatic system and tissues. There is congestion in most of the detoxification channels primarily the kidneys and lymphatic system leading to low immunity and fatigue. This excessive toxicity is affecting the head area and is possibly one of the causes of the ringing in the ears. The pancreas and adrenal gland are weakened and blood sugar is fluctuating. Separation of fibers in the leg areas and an inferior pupil flattening indicate that the legs may be poorly enervated.

Chapter 22

How to take the fear out of going for an iris diagnosis

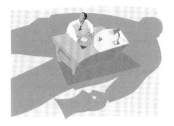

"Knowledge, not fear of the health status of your body gives you the power to overcome any disease that comes your way."

I have chosen this topic because there are still some of you who may be very skeptical or afraid of having your eyes diagnosed. I wanted to use this opportunity to once again reassure those of you who are still unsure, of the many advantages that an iris diagnosis offers and that in the world of alternative medicine, iridologists are no longer placed in the category of charlatans. I will try to answer some of the most frequent questions that I encounter in practice.

Probably the most common response that I hear when an iris diagnosis is offered to a patient is: " **I don't want to know how sick I am.**" Even though patients generally know when something in their bodies is faulty, they don't usually know why. Do you think it is better to pretend that nothing is wrong and wait until something serious happens when you have to seek medical attention? Prevention is always a better option than leaving your health problems to the very last moment. No one wants to spend time in the hospital undergoing all sorts of medical tests, or unnecessary operations that could have been prevented if the condition had been given attention earlier.

People often feel that their health is out of their control. They leave it to their doctors to take care of them when they are ill but do nothing themselves to prevent disease. I feel that the greatest advantage that I offer my patients during an iris diagnosis is an opportunity for them to understand how their body works. They become familiarized with their genetic strengths and weaknesses, so they can make changes in their lifestyle that will improve their health status.

An iris diagnosis does not usually reveal symptoms of a disease but more importantly, it reveals the condition of organs and systems in the body that lead to a disease. In other words, it often provides a tool to find the root of the problem. So much time is wasted these days searching for a diagnosis that would be useful for the patient who has to undergo so many unnecessary and often painful tests as a result. I cannot count the patients I have seen with medical problems for which no one has found a reason.

Unfortunately, those patients have had to visit doctors and specialists and still no one could find the root of their medical problem. Iris diagnosis is not yet a perfect method but what it does offer that classical medical tests do not, is the ability to view each patient individually and to view his or her health status holistically. I believe that the organs in the body all work together in ways that even the greatest experts don't understand. Our body is a miracle. The thousands and thousands of bodily processes that occur every day that we don't even notice and take for granted are remarkable. We cannot just use one faulty organ or one sick part of the body as a basis for our diagnosis. We have to look at every organ and every system because they are all interrelated and one cannot function completely without the other. When I examine the eyes I look at all body systems in order to come up with a diagnosis that takes into account the entire body.

Another frequent question or reaction is: "**I'm healthy, why should I go for an iris diagnosis?**" Again, the important concept to grasp is prevention. An ounce of prevention is worth a pound of cure. Each one of us is born with a genetic iris constitution that has certain strengths and weaknesses and even though we are healthy at present, it doesn't mean we will stay that way. Many of my patients who are in the age between 45 and 55 suddenly experience many health problems all at once and wonder why, since they had been healthy all their lives. The answers lie in the eyes. If they had gone for an iris diagnosis several years earlier, they would have seen those problems in their beginnings, before symptoms had occurred and could have done something then to prevent them from occurring. That is the beauty of iris diagnosis. It is the only method of diagnosis I know that can find problems in the body well before they even become known to the patient as symptoms. Therefore it is just as important for healthy patients to undergo iris diagnosis as it is for sick people.

Another common reaction to iris diagnosis is: "**Iris diagnosis is only for charlatans, how can anyone look at the eyes and diagnose disease?**" For those of you who still have this opinion, I must ask, "what would you trust more, a diagnostic tool that was made by man, or a diagnostic tool made by the ONE who created man?" It is my strong opinion that there is no instrument that man has designed whether it is a computer that analyzes blood, cardiac rhythms, x-rays, or CAT scans, that could even come close to the potential that our own body's eyes can reveal about our health status. This is because the human brain is far more complex than any computer and it is believed that everything that happens to us whether physical or psychological, is registered somewhere in the memory banks of our human computer, the brain. And what is connected through the nervous system to our brain? - our eyes.

I should mention that an iris diagnosis should not replace a classical medical examination but should be used in conjunction to provide additional information on the cause of the patient's disease and as a tool when classical diagnostic methods cannot provide a suitable answer.

Through my studies of thousands of eyes over many years, I have come to one distinct conclusion. There is absolutely no doubt that weaknesses in our body are registered as color changes, marks and signs in the iris, pupil and sclera of the eyes. These signs in the eyes change with our health status. I have seen these changes repeatedly time and time again. I believe that classical medicine will soon have to accept that colors and marks in the eyes change and will have to come up with a reason why. This is happening in many countries in the world today, including America, Australia, Europe, and Russia. So I ask the question once again.

What are you going to believe more, a diagnostic tool designed by man to measure our current state of health, or our wonderful natural organ, the eye, that is connected to our brain and our body every day, every hour, every minute, and every second, recording information on every natural event that occurs in our body?

The study of iridology is no longer for charlatans; it is now a science that although still in its infancy, shows the potential to become the greatest diagnostic tool for medical science. As modern medicine further moves in the direction of specialization, alternative medicine is moving back to viewing each individual as a whole unique organism where each system in the body is dependent and interrelated to the other.

The final question that patients should ask is: **" How do we know if a health professional is properly qualified to do an iris diagnosis?"** Ask to see a diploma in natural medicine where iridology has been studied from an accredited school or university. Ask how long the iridologist has been using iridology with patients as experience is worth its weight in gold. Ask what equipment the iridologist uses for iris diagnosis. Many iridologists use only a magnifying glass and it is my decided opinion that there is no way that an accurate diagnosis can be performed with a magnifying glass alone, as the patients will get only a superficial diagnosis.

The eyes should be photographed with a special microscope camera and then the photos intensely analyzed so that every mark is measured properly. The best way today is by use of computer technology. Ask for a copy of the pictures of your eyes and a thorough written analysis. A competent, experienced iridologist who knows what he is doing will provide all of the above.

Perhaps, sometime in this new millennium, we shall gain the strength and courage to believe in our own bodies and begin to accept new natural methods of diagnosis, such as iris diagnosis, and begin to use natural methods to cure, rather than drugs. Perhaps we will have to because we are not machines and the irresponsible use of drugs is damaging our physical and mental health. On one hand we look down on those who are addicted to drugs such as heroin while at the same time we swallow pills every time we have a headache, every time we are constipated, every time we have an allergy, and every time our stomach is upset. Ask yourselves, "Who is the drug addict?" We are a part of nature and our health depends on how natural the nutrients that we ingest are. We eventually pay the price for our unnatural way of life.

Perhaps the greatest fear you should have when you go for an iris diagnosis is that you may have to come to the realization that no doctor or no drug is going to cure your chronic disease and that the only effective way to improve your health status is by making responsible lifestyle changes.

Chapter 23

Conclusion: Change, harmony, iris diagnosis, and mankind's search for a return to health

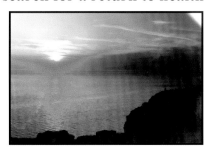

"I believe that the world is changing. People are changing. People are searching for a greater fulfillment. We will look to the past as a primitive time. War, money, drugs, greed, power, racism. These are primitive words. Words of the second millennium. Cooperation, exchange of ideas, common goals, respect for nature, equality and natural medicine are words of the third millennium, the new millennium."

Often the greatest scientific discoveries in the past have initially received the most opposition and criticism from skeptics. Alternative medicine is no exception. Despite its use for thousands of years around the world, somehow in the last few hundred years we have put natural forms of healing aside, and in our quest for quick-acting cures we have opted for much easier methods using drugs and chemical preparations. As I hope I have adequately expressed in this book, this is not the future answer to our growing medical problems. Fortunately, alternative medicine and iris diagnosis have survived through the ages and today there is renewed excitement and growing interest in these methods. The time has come for change.

Mankind always seems to have a defensive reaction to change in the way we do things. We find it very difficult to accept change. We especially see it in the older generation who have been used to doing a task a certain way for years and years. We see it in the medical profession, in their cries against natural and alternative medicine despite its growing success around the world. We see it in ourselves, as we are often unprepared to change our lifestyle habits and diet to achieve better health. People feel threatened by a new way of thinking. For the insecure person, change often evokes a negative reaction in the form of stubborn attempts to block it out of mind and to fight against it. For the individual with an open mind however, change is welcomed as it stimulates and challenges learning. Remember, a closed mind learns nothing new. If we are going to advance as a society in the reduction of sickness and disease, we must be prepared for and be open to change.

Nature's laws cannot be abused. We cannot act like gods and influence our health and our bodies through unnatural methods. The body will always respond in a negative way. The body has its natural processes of repair and regeneration and needs natural nutrients to carry them out. We cannot fool our bodies, only ourselves. You see, our body, mind, and spirit are in harmony with nature and the world around us. Any slight upset to this intricate homeostasis, and our physical, mental, and spiritual health status is drastically affected. We are only now, starting to learn about holistic health.

Iris diagnosis is in my opinion one of the best means available to learn about holistic health and the health status of the body. It reveals the damaging effects that drugs, chemicals, and unnatural lifestyle habits have on our organs and systems, while at the same time, it provides a means to view positive changes when we start living and eating in more healthy ways. It is a branch of alternative medicine that has helped thousands and thousands of patients around the world to find the cause of their disease and to monitor changes on their return to health.

What do we want out of our lives? Generally when I ask my patients if they would like to live to 120 years or more like some of the mighty Hunza people, they say they would not. Why? Because most people see old age as a time when one is in and out of the hospital, when one is neglected by family and friends, when one no longer has a purpose in life and is often a burden on others. I am sure that if we were given reassurance that we would remain healthy and happy to the age of 150 years, most of us would choose to live that long. If we are strong and healthy we will not be a burden on others, we will be able to contribute to society even to an old age, and will have time to share our lives and experiences with our children, grandchildren, and great grandchildren.

What are we prepared to invest for our health? While most of us will invest thousands of dollars into real estate, business, our careers, stocks, bonds and lottery tickets, our health is usually on the bottom of the list. Most of us are also unaware that we spend an unbelievable amount of money on headache, flu and cold preparations, laxatives, anti-histamines, antibiotics, and other drugs for our day- to- day ailments which temporarily ease our symptoms, but do very little in treating the cause. Sooner or later these problems will worsen until they manifest themselves as serious health conditions.

What are the rewards of achieving optimum health? More energy to achieve things in life, and a clear, healthy, happy, and peaceful mind that will be open to learning and enjoying all that life brings us. What use is a pile of money or investments when we cannot enjoy them due to poor health? We all know this, but often remember only, when a serious disease like cancer, heart disease or diabetes overcomes us. We must learn to invest in preventative medicine. One of the best methods of practicing preventative medicine is iris diagnosis combined with diet and lifestyle changes. I have included a list in this book of what I believe are some of the most important diet and lifestyle changes that we can make to optimize our health.

Remember we are all individuals, with specific needs to maintain health. Like each one of our irises, none of us is the same. We need to learn about our individual health status, what genetic constitution we belong to and what the current condition of the organs and systems in our bodies is. We will then be equipped with information that can assist us in terms of what nutrients we are deficient in and what nutrients can improve our state of health.

What lies ahead in the future? I don't have a crystal ball to look into, but I believe the future of alternative medicine or medicine for that matter must include viewing the body holistically. I believe in order to cure disease the doctors of the future will not be able to use primitive methods like drugs or chemicals but will have to assist the body's natural processes of regeneration by taking all aspects of human health into consideration, and using only natural methods. This means that even the psychological and spiritual effects on the body will have to be considered as well. Some natural therapists who deal with cancer and degenerative disease, already believe that the cause is psychological, often due to psychological trauma or prolonged mental suffering that taxes the body and places it in a nutrient- deficient state much like that of stress. It may therefore be unnecessary to remove a tumor or use radiation therapy or chemotherapy as the root of the problem must be found if inner healing is to be accomplished. The body as mentioned before, has amazing capabilities to regenerate itself if given the right natural nutrients in the right amounts. Diseases cannot form, when the body is in optimum health.

I believe that in time, diagnosis from the eyes or iris diagnosis will become a leading natural method for finding the cause of disease and for monitoring health status changes.

I thank all of you who have embarked upon this journey of change with me, into the world of iris diagnosis, in order to gain a new perspective on health and the diagnosis of disease.

I hope that this book has provided a greater understanding of the science and art of iridology as well as an inspiration to lead a healthier life.

Wishing you the best of natural health.
I'll be keeping an eye on you.

Frank Navratil BSc. N.D.

FRANK NAVRATIL'S LIST OF DIET AND LIFESTYLE CHANGES FOR A LONG AND HEALTHY LIFE

1. **CHOOSE WATER** instead of alcohol, beer, wine, coffee or tea - minimum 1-2 liters/day.
2. **DRINK JUICE** that is pure 100% with no added sugar and dilute with water 50%.
3. **SKIP DESSERTS** and have fruit, dates, figs, or raisins instead.
4. **EAT 5 SMALLER MEALS** instead of 3 large ones (breakfast, 10:30, lunch, 3:30, dinner).
5. **CUT OUT DAIRY PRODUCTS** (milk, soft cheese, cream, ice cream) you can get calcium from much better sources like green vegetables, almonds, avocados, and sesame seeds
6. **NO EXTRA ADDED SALT**
7. **LESS PACKAGED, TINNED, AND FROZEN FOODS -** go for fresh!
8. **EAT NATURAL WHITE YOGURTS ONLY** with no added sugar, skim milk powder, or cream.
9. **COOK FOOD MINIMALLY -** no microwave
10. **DO NOT FRY FOODS -** bake, steam, or boil
11. **EAT 25% MEAT and 75 % VEGETABLES**
12. **EAT FISH** 3-4 times per week (especially those high in Omega 3 fatty acids – like salmon and tuna)
13. **EAT WHOLEGRAIN** pastas, rice, and wholegrain breads - no white bread
14. **AT RESTAURANTS** order food without gravies, and more fish instead of red meat
15. **EAT POTATOES MINIMALLY -** too many potatoes leave no room for the 75% vegetables
16. **DO NOT USE MARGARINES / ARTIFICIAL SPREADS -** butter is more natural but not too much
17. **EAT A FRESH SALAD EVERY DAY** - include broccoli, celery, bean sprouts, green beans, alfalfa, carrots, cucumber, green peppers, and others and use toppings like olive oil or fresh lemon juice and herbs for seasoning.
18. **EAT NUTS AND SEEDS,** especially almonds, sunflower seeds and sesame seeds.
19. **EAT A VARIETY OF FRUIT** that is fresh, not cooked, canned, or frozen
20. **USE SPICES** rather than sauces, gravies or artificial toppings
21. **DRINK HERBAL TEAS** with no sugar
22. **DO NOT USE ARTIFICIAL SWEETENERS**
23. **ALWAYS BUY FOOD WITHOUT PRESERVATIVES, ADDED COLOURS OR CHEMICALS**
24. **EXERCISE** 30- 60 minutes 3-5 times per week
25. **FIND EXERCISE YOU ENJOY** like sports, walking, bike riding, swimming, aerobics
26. **CARRY HEALTHY FOOD WITH YOU** so you are not tempted to buy junk food
27. **RELAX** at least half an hour every day - meditate, listen to music etc.
28. **DEEP BREATHING** five minutes every day
29. **REMIND YOURSELF** to take things easy - don't worry over things you can't change

30. **SPEND SOME TIME IN NATURE** – every day whether it's a walk through the park.....
31. **DO 1 NICE THING** for someone every day without asking for anything in return
32. **SMILE** at least 5 times a day at someone
33. **FREE ANY NEGATIVE EMOTIONS** like grief, anger, distrust and jealousy
34. **ACCEPT AND BE HAPPY** with who you are and with your journey in life
35. **LISTEN TO YOUR INTUITION** and let it guide you along your path in life
36. **FIND A BALANCE** between work, family, friends, hobbies and interests
37. **TAKE CONTROL OF YOUR OWN HEALTH!** Use natural forms of noninvasive diagnostic methods like iris diagnosis and use only natural drug-free healing methods
38. **TAKE NATURAL VITAMINS AND SUPPLEMENTS** to assist your weak organs to heal themselves
39. **AIM FOR 80% COMPLIANCE** with the above – 100% is impossible and we are not perfect!

RETURN TO HEALTH

NATUROPATHIC CLINIC

IRIS DIAGNOSIS, BOWEN THERAPY, NATUROPATHY

MAKE AN APPOINTMENT WITH FRANK NAVRATIL BSc. N.D.

IN THE CZECH REPUBLIC

For:

IRIS DIAGNOSIS

BOWEN THERAPY

NATURAL VITAMIN AND MINERAL THERAPY

NATUROPATHY

Email: frank.navratil@volny.cz

Visit my personal web sites for more information

www.volny.cz/frank.navratil

OR

www.irisdiagnosis.net

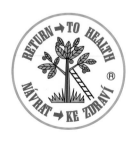

RETURN TO HEALTH

INTERNET MAGAZINE

www.navratkezdravi.cz

THE FIRST CZECH/ENGLISH INTERNET MAGAZINE SOLELY DEVOTED TO ALTERNATIVE MEDICINE

ARTICLES WRITTEN BY LEADING HEALERS HERE AND OVERSEAS

Articles on:

Alternative diagnostic methods

Alternative diets

Ingestive therapy, vitamins, herbal medicine

Holistic healing methods

Exercise and movement therapies

Healing methods associated with our senses

Healing with touch and life energy

Psychological healing methods

Other healing methods

Healthy recipes

Information including books about alternative medicine, courses, events, health products, explanations of alternative medicine methods, and contacts for healers.

www.navratkezdravi.cz

RETURN TO HEALTH

COURSES

IRISDIAGNOSIS / BOWEN METHOD

IRISDIAGNOSIS 1,2,3, NUTRITION FOR IRIDOLOGISTS

INTRODUCTORY, INTERMEDIATE AND ADVANCED COURSES ON IRIS DIAGNOSIS AND NUTRITION

CORRESPONDENCE CD ROM

BOWEN METHOD

COURSE IN THE BOWEN METHOD OF PRESSURE THERAPY

FOR MORE INFORMATION ON COURSES:

Email: frank.navratil@volny.cz

PLEASE VISIT MY PERSONAL WEB SITES FOR MORE INFORMATION ON COURSES

www.volny.cz/frank.navratil

Or

www.irisdiagnosis.net

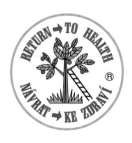

RETURN TO HEALTH

HEALTH BOOKS

IF YOU HAVE ENJOYED THIS BOOK BY FRANK NAVRATIL BSc. N.D. THEN PLEASE LOOK FOR HIS NEW BOOK WHICH WILL BE AVAILABLE SOON AND ENTITLED:

"THE EYE FOR AN EYE DIET"

NUTRITION AND HEALTH BY GENETIC IRIS CONSTITUTION

INFORMATION CAN BE OBTAINED FROM:

Email: frank.navratil@volny.cz

OR VISIT MY WEB SITES:

www.volny.cz/frank.navratil

Or

www.irisdiagnosis.net

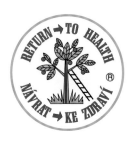

RETURN TO HEALTH

IRIS DIAGNOSIS PRODUCTS

IRIS CHARTS / IRIS FLASH CARDS/ MAGNIFYING LENSES / SELF-ANALYSIS MIRRORS
IRIS DIAGNOSIS COMPUTER PROGRAMS / COMPLETE IRIDOLOGY DIGITAL CAPTURE
AND ANALYSIS SYSTEMS

IRIS CHARTS

FULL COLOUR LAMINATED IRIS MAPS BY FRANK NAVRATIL
BSc. N.D.

IRIS FLASH CARDS

FULL COLOUR FUNDAMENTAL IRIS SIGNS WITH EXPLANATIONS

MAGNIFYING LENSES

GERMAN-MADE LENS (10x) WITH ADJUSTABLE KRYPTON LIGHT

SELF-ANALYSIS MIRRORS

A UNIQUE MIRRORED LENS AND LIGHT THAT ALLOWS YOU TO
ANALYZE YOUR OWN EYES

IRIS DIAGNOSTIC EQUIPMENT, PROGRAMS,
AND FULL SYSTEMS

ADVANCED PRODUCTS FOR THE SERIOUS IRIDOLOGIST

FOR PRICES AND MORE INFORMATION:

Email: frank.navratil@volny.cz

or see our web sites:

www.volny.cz/frank.navratil

Or

www.irisdiagnosis.net